Milady Standard Esthetics: Fundamentals Exam Review

Eleventh Edition

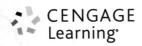

CENGAGE
Learning·

Australia • Brazil • Japan • Korea • Mexico • Singapore • Spain • United Kingdom • United States

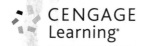

CENGAGE
Learning®

Milady Standard Esthetics:
Fundamentals Exam Review,
Eleventh Edition
Milady

President, Milady:
Dawn Gerrain

Director of Content and
Business Development:
Sandra Bruce

Acquisitions Editor:
Martine Edwards

Associate Acquisitions Editor:
Philip Mandl

Senior Product Manager:
Jessica Mahoney

Director of Marketing and
Training:
Gerard McAvey

Senior Production Director:
Wendy A. Troeger

Production Manager:
Sherondra Thedford

Senior Content Project
Manager:
Nina Tucciarelli

Technology Director:
Sandy Charette

Senior Art Director:
Benjamin Gleeksman

For product information and technology assistance, contact us at
Professional & Career Group Customer Support,
1-800-648-7450
For permission to use material from this text or product,
submit all requests online at **cengage.com/permissions.**
Further permissions questions can be e-mailed to
permissionrequest@cengage.com.

Library of Congress Control Number: 2011943910

ISBN-13: 9781111306922

ISBN-10: 1111306923

Milady
5 Maxwell Drive
Clifton Park, NY 12065-2919
USA

Cengage Learning products are represented in Canada by Nelson Education, Ltd.

For your lifelong learning solutions, visit **milady.cengage.com**

Visit our corporate website at **cengage.com.**

Printed in United States of America
1 2 3 4 5 XX 16 15 14 13 12

Milady Standard Esthetics: Fundamentals Exam Review

Foreword

Milady Standard Esthetics: Fundamentals Exam Review has been revised to follow the type of skin care questions most frequently used by states and by the national testing, conducted under the auspices of the National-Interstate Council of State Boards of Cosmetology.

This review book is designed to be of major assistance to students in preparing for the state license examinations. The exclusive concentration on multiple-choice test items reflects the fact that all state board examinations and national testing examinations are confined to this type of question.

Questions on the state board examinations in different states will not be exactly like these and may not touch upon all the information covered in this review. However, students who diligently study and practice their work as taught in the classroom and who use this book for test preparation and review should receive higher grades on both classroom and license examinations.

Part 1: Orientation

CHAPTER 1—HISTORY AND CAREER OPPORTUNITIES IN ESTHETICS

1. Who is responsible for examinations, licensing, and standards?
   a. state licensing inspectors
   b. state board members
   c. licensing specialists
   d. esthetician examiners   ____

2. What did the ancient Egyptians do before other cultures?
   a. cultivate beauty in an extravagant fashion
   b. build magnificent public baths
   c. develop the hair-removal practice of threading
   d. develop cosmetic surgery   ____

3. What is restoration work?
   a. surgical procedures used to help rebuild bodies after accidents
   b. another name for cosmetic surgery
   c. the esthetics specialization associated with mortuary science
   d. rebuilding hairstyles after a long day   ____

4. Why were the ancient Hebrews able to adopt many skin care and grooming techniques from other cultures?
   a. their level of education was higher than that of other cultures
   b. they were nomadic
   c. they cultivated a sense of what we now call "the global community"
   d. they were entrepreneurial   ____

5. What is a dye derived from leaves and shoots of the mignonette tree?
   a. elderberry
   b. henna
   c. camilla
   d. pomegranate   ____

6. What type of magnificent public buildings were the ancient Romans famous for constructing?
   a. smokehouses
   b. baths
   c. swimming pools
   d. massage parlors   ____

7. What is the primary purpose of camouflage makeup?
   a. to disguise imperfections such as scars
   b. to create the illusion that someone has darker skin than they do
   c. to shield the skin from the harmful effects of the sun
   d. to make a person stand out in public   ____

8. Where was the ancient method of hair removal known as threading invented?
   - a. Vietnam
   - b. Korea
   - c. China
   - d. Japan

   _____

9. What is the ancient Greek word meaning "skilled in the use of cosmetics"?
   - a. *kozmetikos*
   - b. *cosmetticoso*
   - c. *kazamattika*
   - d. *cosomotico*

   _____

10. Where on their faces did women wear colored makeup during the Middle Ages?
    - a. eyes and lips
    - b. cheeks and lips
    - c. eyes and nose
    - d. nose and cheeks

    _____

11. What does a manufacturer's representative do?
    - a. train others on product knowledge and how to sell products
    - b. perform safety inspections
    - c. sell products to customers
    - d. perform esthetics treatments on clients

    _____

12. What was a bare (shaved or tweezed) eyebrow thought to signify during the Renaissance?
    - a. greater social standing
    - b. greater wealth
    - c. greater intelligence
    - d. greater fertility

    _____

13. What do mobile estheticians do?
    - a. move from station to station within the salon
    - b. own portable equipment and make house or office calls
    - c. rotate between several different salons within a chain
    - d. work at two or more independently-owned salons

    _____

14. What was true of some elaborate hairstyles during the Age of Extravagance?
    - a. they contained fountains with running water
    - b. they contained gardens and menageries
    - c. they contained elaborate electrical light effects
    - d. they featured movement created by the use of hydraulics

    _____

15. What is product development?
    - a. amount of time a product needs to cure before it can be used
    - b. practice of getting clients accustomed to certain products
    - c. field of creating new products and technologies
    - d. practice of building a customer base for a new product

    _____

16. When did women pinch their cheeks and bite their lips to add color?
    a. Age of Extravagance   c. Victorian Age
    b. Elizabethan Era   d. Renaissance   _____

17. What career should those with journalistic abilities consider pursuing?
    a. state licensing inspector   c. esthetics writer
    b. esthetics educator   d. state board member   _____

18. What is a buyer's responsibility?
    a. demonstrating the use of products to salon managers and
       estheticians
    b. making "secret shopper" visits to ensure stores are not
       overcharging
    c. purchasing products from one store to resell them in another
    d. purchasing products to be sold and used in stores   _____

19. What term refers to the art of manipulating materials on an
    atomic or molecular scale?
    a. nucleotechnology   c. nanotechnology
    b. minitechnology   d. microtechnology   _____

20. Who visits spas and salons to ensure compliance with state
    regulations?
    a. official state spa technician
    b. state licensing inspector
    c. state cosmetics regulator
    d. official state esthetician   _____

21. What did the ancient Egyptians use to dye hair and tattoo skin?
    a. henna   c. animal blood
    b. rosemary   d. crushed stone   _____

22. What term refers to a profession that integrates surgical
    procedures with esthetic treatments?
    a. cosmetology   c. medical aesthetician
    b. beauty technician   d. makeup stylist   _____

23. When did women use bleach to make their hair blond?
    a. Renaissance   c. age of the Roman Empire
    b. Middle Ages   d. age of the ancient Greeks _____

24. What became a common practice in the twentieth century?
    a. creating elaborate hairstyles featuring gardens and menageries
    b. creating body art with henna
    c. dyeing the hair blond with bleach
    d. cosmetic surgery   _____

25. What ancient culture commonly offered physical treatments in public baths?
    a. Greek   c. Japanese
    b. Hebrew   d. Roman   _____

26. When did a more relaxed approach to clothing, hair, and makeup become popular?
    a. beginning of the twenty-first century
    b. middle of the eighteenth century
    c. end of the nineteenth century
    d. beginning of the twentieth century   _____

27. What ancient culture used the way a person looked naked as the basis for determining beauty?
    a. Greek   c. Japanese
    b. Roman   d. Chinese   _____

28. Who issues requests for compounding pharmacies to mix special preparations?
    a. physicians
    b. nurses
    c. salon managers
    d. manufacturer's representatives   _____

29. What did the ancient Hebrews use to moisten and protect the skin?
    a. olive and grapeseed oils c. rosemary and thyme
    b. henna   d. mineral water   _____

30. What can estheticians do if they obtain a medical license?
    a. dispense drugs in the salon
    b. prescribe medications
    c. formulate and sell medications
    d. perform surgery in the salon   _____

31. What must you obtain before you become an esthetics educator?
    a. medical license   c. doctorate degree
    b. master's degree   d. certification   _____

32. What type of esthetics work requires that you join a union?
    a. booth rental
    b. mobile esthetician
    c. manufacturer's representative
    d. film and TV makeup artist   _____

33. What should you know before deciding to become a cosmetics buyer?
   a. you must receive certification before becoming a buyer
   b. you will travel a great deal if you become a buyer
   c. you will spend most of your time alone if you become a buyer
   d. you will rarely interact with new people if you become a buyer   ____

34. What type of esthetics work requires the supervision of a mortician?
   a. restoration
   b. revivification
   c. reconstitution
   d. recombination   ____

35. What is a career that requires an outgoing personality for success?
   a. restoration makeup worker
   b. state licensing inspector
   c. esthetics writer
   d. manufacturer's representative   ____

CHAPTER 2—LIFE SKILLS

1. What term refers to the conscious act of planning your life?
   a. game plan
   b. personal scheme
   c. life design
   d. course of action
   ____

2. What propels you to do something?
   a. procrastination
   b. motivation
   c. criticism
   d. self-management
   ____

3. When you prioritize, in what order should you list tasks that need to be done?
   a. most to least important
   b. least to most important
   c. easiest to hardest
   d. hardest to easiest
   ____

4. What do good life skills help you achieve?
   a. guaranteed financial success
   b. your personal best
   c. guaranteed career advancement
   d. more than anyone else
   ____

5. What is your professional responsibility with regard to personal problems?
   a. seek guidance from your manager
   b. seek guidance from your clients
   c. keep these problems to yourself
   d. avoid people when you're in a bad mood
   ____

6. What helps you understand the needs and desires of the people around you?
   a. judgment
   b. communication
   c. prioritizing
   d. self-management
   ____

7. What is true about deep breathing?
   a. it is an effective tool for stress management
   b. it should be avoided in the workplace because of chemicals
   c. you should only do this after work because you need time to relax
   d. it is relaxing, but it inhibits your concentration
   ____

8. When should you begin organizing for the next day?
   a. at the end of the work day
   b. during your last appointment
   c. while you are having lunch
   d. whenever you take a break
   ____

9. What is time management?
   a. allotting time for tasks so all tasks can be completed
   b. making a list of things you want to accomplish
   c. keeping track of what time it is throughout the day
   d. supervising people to make sure they record their time properly _____

10. What is your scope of practice?
   a. the hours your salon is open every day
   b. the amount of time you can make available to each client
   c. the geographical region in which you can legally operate
   d. the products and treatments you can offer _____

11. What is teamwork?
   a. working collaboratively to maintain productivity and reduce stress
   b. helping others do their jobs even if you have a client at your station
   c. identifying tasks that your supervisor can perform for you
   d. asking other estheticians to help you perform client services _____

12. What term refers to putting off until tomorrow what you can do today?
   a. time management   c. prioritizing
   b. scheduling   d. procrastination _____

13. What does a mission statement establish?
   a. how much money a business will make in its first year
   b. the values an institution or individual lives by
   c. how many employees a business will have after five years
   d. which charities a business plans to support _____

14. What is **NOT** an element of a good work ethic?
   a. trustworthiness   c. respectfulness
   b. tardiness   d. supportiveness _____

15. What are boundaries?
   a. limits you set on sharing personal information
   b. physical borders of your work station
   c. draping you place across clients to protect them from spillage
   d. limits you set on how much work you are willing to do _____

16. What is the term for your outlook on life, based on your beliefs?
   a. attitude   c. equilibrium
   b. emotional stability   d. reliability _____

17. What is **NOT** one of the things that will determine your success?
    a. the way you handle yourself
    b. your technical skills
    c. whether you get a medical license
    d. the way you behave toward others   ____

18. What is a good strategy if you find studying overwhelming?
    a. break studying down into manageable tasks
    b. cram at the end so you get studying over with quickly
    c. learn everything you can during class and avoid studying
    d. find out what is on the exam and learn only that information   ____

19. What posture should you use when studying?
    a. lying down on your back
    b. lying down on your chest
    c. sitting upright
    d. sitting in a reclining position   ____

20. What is true about mission statements?
    a. they are essential elements of business plans
    b. they are optional elements of business plans
    c. they should not be created until the business is already
       operating
    d. mission statements are not appropriate for every business   ____

21. What helps you decide what you want out of life?
    a. procrastinating   c. time management
    b. goal setting   d. prioritizing   ____

22. What does the term *ethics* refer to?
    a. moral principles by which we live and work
    b. laws that keep us from stealing from employers
    c. regulations that state which products can be used
    d. services you can perform, based on your certification   ____

23. Why should you learn from your mistakes?
    a. so you know how to get away with things in the workplace
    b. so you know the limitations of your abilities
    c. to help you grow in your professional life
    d. to help you avoid interactions with your manager   ____

24. What blocks the creative mind from exploring ideas?
    a. feedback   c. criticism
    b. guidance   d. enthusiasm   ____

25. What term refers to a well thought-out process for achieving something?
    a. self-management   c. prioritizing
    b. procrastination   d. time management   ____

26. What is diplomacy?
    a. keeping personal problems to yourself
    b. being tactful in your dealings with others
    c. making critical observations when people do things wrong
    d. telling a client she looks good when she actually does not   ____

27. What is true of a pleasing attitude?
    a. it will gain you associates, clients, and friends
    b. it will send the message you can be pushed around by managers
    c. it makes clients worry that you will only say what they want to hear
    d. it will benefit you in your private life, but not in your work life   ____

28. What is true about obtaining appropriate state licensure or certification?
    a. it is not necessary for establishing credibility as an esthetician
    b. it is the first step to establishing credibility as an esthetician
    c. only managers are expected to have licenses and certificates
    d. only salon owners are expected to have licenses and certificates   ____

29. What is true about staying on time with appointments?
    a. it is not very important, because clients are almost always late
    b. it is a minor aspect of time management for estheticians
    c. it is the most important aspect of time management for estheticians
    d. you should expect to fall behind at least once every day   ____

30. How early should a new client arrive before his or her first appointment in order to fill out a client intake form?
    a. 5 to 10 minutes   c. 15 to 30 minutes
    b. 10 to 15 minutes   d. 30 to 45 minutes   ____

10

31. How should you measure your sense of achievement?
    a. by asking other people whether they consider you successful
    b. by comparing your achievements to your definition of success
    c. by keeping track of how much money your fellow students make
    d. by comparing your achievements to your parents' level of affluence _____

32. What is true of a healthy lifestyle?
    a. it is a tremendous asset in reaching your goals
    b. it is a luxury for people with money to buy gym memberships
    c. it has no bearing upon your professional career
    d. it is impossible to live a healthy lifestyle if you are an esthetician _____

33. What will happen if you demonstrate good manners?
    a. you will get along with every single person you meet
    b. you will engender goodwill and respect
    c. you will never have problems with your clients or managers
    d. you will always earn larger tips than other estheticians in your salon _____

34. When should you ask questions in class?
    a. when you don't understand something
    b. when you want to give the impression you are paying attention
    c. whenever the teacher discusses something you find interesting
    d. whenever the teacher discusses what information will be on the exam _____

CHAPTER 3—YOUR PROFESSIONAL IMAGE

1. When choosing makeup for work, what should be your first priority?
   a. making yourself look seductive
   b. accentuating your best features
   c. making yourself look glamorous
   d. showing off your makeup skills   ____

2. How much time of the relaxation response can one exercise session generate?
   a. 10 minutes   c. two hours
   b. 30 minutes   d. eight hours   ____

3. What affects your interaction with everyone in the salon?
   a. your activities outside work   c. your technical skills
   b. your professional image   d. your level of education   ____

4. What is **NOT** an aspect of your professional conduct?
   a. how you get along with clients
   b. how you get along with co-workers
   c. how you behave in the workplace
   d. how you dress in the workplace   ____

5. What term refers to the impression you project, informed by your appearance, attitude, and abilities?
   a. personal conduct   c. professional conduct
   b. personal image   d. professional image   ____

6. What is the purpose of the makeup you wear at work?
   a. displaying healthy, beautiful skin
   b. advertising "hot" new products
   c. making you look attractive
   d. color coordinating with clothes   ____

7. What is an element of good standing posture?
   a. keeping your back arched   c. leaning forward
   b. keeping your back straight   d. leaning backward   ____

8. What should you do if you have long hair and work as an esthetician?
   a. cut it to a more manageable length
   b. wear it down to show clients you understand beauty
   c. wear it swept up and off the shoulders
   d. wear it in a long braid down your back   ____

9. What can you do to avoid scratching clients' skin?
   a. wear gloves so your fingernails don't touch the client's skin
   b. avoid letting your fingertips touch the client's skin
   c. soak your fingernails in solvents that make fingernails soft
   d. keep your fingernails from getting too long _____

10. What is **NOT** an aspect of personal hygiene?
    a. freshening up throughout the day as necessary
    b. brushing and flossing your teeth
    c. using deodorant
    d. wearing strongly scented perfume _____

11. What is the term for posture that is healthy for the spine?
    a. ergonomically correct   c. osteospinally correct
    b. cardiovertabraically correct   d. endemically correct _____

12. What should your image impress on the minds of your clients?
    a. intimidate them
    b. earn their trust
    c. show that you are willing to do whatever is asked of you
    d. create a sense of mystery _____

13. How will you spend a lot of time as an esthetician?
    a. leaning against a wall and sitting on a stool
    b. standing on your feet and lying down
    c. standing on your feet and sitting on a stool
    d. sitting on the floor and lying on a treatment table _____

14. When should you count to 10 and think before you speak?
    a. when conflicts arise
    b. whenever you speak with your manager
    c. whenever you speak with a client
    d. at all times _____

15. How can you convey an image of confidence?
    a. by sitting quietly and alone
    b. by practicing good posture
    c. by speaking very loudly
    d. by offering opinions on everything _____

16. What makes clients eager for your knowledge?
    a. your good professional image
    b. the certification on your wall
    c. the way your work station looks
    d. how attractive you are _____

17. What sort of fragrances are **NEVER** appropriate for the workplace?
    a. heavy
    b. subtle
    c. floral
    d. fruity
    ____

18. What is true about exposed undergarments?
    a. they make a strong fashion statement in the workplace
    b. they add a sense of sexiness to the workplace
    c. they are never appropriate in the workplace
    d. they are occasionally appropriate in the workplace
    ____

19. What should you save for after business hours?
    a. subtle makeup that accentuates your best features
    b. trendy looks such as heavily made-up eyes and black nail polish
    c. clean, comfortable clothes that are fashionable but not overtly sexy
    d. simple jewelry, like stud earrings, that do not make a lot of noise
    ____

20. What are three important elements of physical presentation?
    a. posture, walk, movements
    b. clothing, hair, jewelry
    c. shoes, accessories, makeup
    d. muscle tone, tan, cleavage
    ____

21. How can you make your clients confident in your ability to help them?
    a. by using fancy industry jargon and dropping cool brand names
    b. by following your own advice and practicing good skin care
    c. by talking about the way celebrities do their makeup
    d. by pointing out how good other estheticians in the salon look
    ____

22. What is true of daily bathing or showering?
    a. it is not an expectation for professional estheticians
    b. daily bathing or showering is one of the basics of personal hygiene
    c. it is only recommended when the weather is extremely humid
    d. for estheticians, several showers per day are recommended
    ____

23. Why should you check your salon's policy before picking a fragrance you intend to wear in the workplace?
    a. to make sure your salon manager is not allergic to the fragrance
    b. most salons require that estheticians wear heavy fragrances
    c. many salons have a no-fragrance policy
    d. to make sure none of your clients is allergic to the fragrance
    ____

24. What is a danger posed by defective body postures?
    a. physical problems   c. awkward socialization
    b. wardrobe malfunctions   d. fashion faux pas   _____

25. What do you exhibit when you keep the soles of your feet entirely on the floor while seated?
    a. social discomfort
    b. proper sitting posture
    c. unprofessional appearance
    d. distended tendon syndrome   _____

26. What do you do when you refrain from criticism?
    a. take the high road
    b. take the low road
    c. give the impression you are weak
    d. miss opportunities for advancement   _____

27. What begins with, and stays grounded in, health?
    a. self-centeredness   c. sexual attractiveness
    b. personal confidence   d. real beauty   _____

28. What can eating a nutritious diet help you achieve?
    a. success   c. popularity
    b. balance   d. perfect skin   _____

29. What is a good description of the clothing you should wear in the workplace?
    a. formless and loose   c. fashionable and sexy
    b. broken-in and comfortable d. clean and fresh   _____

30. When are open-toed shoes appropriate for work?
    a. on hot days   c. anytime
    b. on humid days   d. never   _____

31. What is a desirable characteristic of the socks or hosiery you wear at work?
    a. fashionably frayed
    b. contrast with your attire
    c. different color on each leg
    d. free of runs   _____

32. What should you do when conflicts arise?
    a. get another opinion before making a judgment
    b. ask your manager to resolve all conflicts for you
    c. provide examples to support your point of view
    d. assume you are at fault and submit your resignation   _____

33. What is an important aspect of maintaining good standing posture?
    a. tilting your head toward your dominant side
    b. pulling your abdomen in so that it is flat
    c. keeping your knees locked
    d. keeping your neck scrunched up toward your shoulders _____

34. What enables you to make the right choices for yourself?
    a. achieving balance   c. becoming popular
    b. becoming successful   d. receiving a degree _____

CHAPTER 4—COMMUNICATING FOR SUCCESS

1. What do you earn when you approach a new client with a smile on your face?
   a. a new personal friendship
   b. trust and loyalty
   c. a bonus from your manager
   d. career advancement _____

2. When should a client fill out an intake form?
   a. before arriving at the salon
   b. before receiving services
   c. during treatment
   d. after treatment _____

3. What is considered a legal document?
   a. intake form
   b. color chart
   c. consent form
   d. service record _____

4. Why should you offer a compliment if you see that a co-worker has done something well?
   a. that's the only way to get a compliment in return
   b. so your manager will see you praising a co-worker
   c. managers are too busy to keep up employee morale
   d. everyone benefits from a well-deserved compliment _____

5. What does everyone in the salon deserve from you?
   a. respect
   b. assistance with their jobs
   c. personal favors
   d. affection _____

6. What is an appropriate action in the event of unethical behavior on the part of the manager, such as sexual harassment or misappropriating funds?
   a. perform a citizen's arrest
   b. challenge the manager's authority
   c. physically eject the manager from the salon
   d. create a petition demanding the manager's termination _____

7. What is an example of a positive nonverbal cue?
   a. checking out your nails while someone is talking
   b. yawning during conversation
   c. good eye contact
   d. looking at your shoes while someone is talking _____

8. When should you make amends?
   a. when you can tell the manager dislikes something you did
   b. when you are wrong
   c. when you can tell a co-worker dislikes something you did
   d. you never need to make amends ____

9. What must you master in order to thrive in the field of aesthetics?
   a. psychology
   b. psychiatry
   c. the art of manipulation
   d. the art of communication ____

10. What is based on trust?
    a. your scope of practice
    b. strong professional relationships
    c. certification and licensure
    d. your personal satisfaction ____

11. How can you ensure continued patronage from your clients?
    a. by saying you're the only person who can make them look good
    b. by perfecting professional communication
    c. by perfecting professional manipulation
    d. by giving clients free samples every time they visit the salon ____

12. When should a client be asked to reschedule his or her appointment?
    a. when he or she arrives more than 15 minutes late
    b. when you're not in the mood to interact with that particular client
    c. when you can tell the client is in a rotten mood
    d. when he or she arrives more then five minutes late ____

13. What is a good description of a client who should be scheduled at the end of the day?
    a. someone who his habitually late
    b. someone who is never sure of the services they want
    c. someone who is often rude to the salon staff
    d. someone who is habitually talkative ____

14. When should you argue with a client?
    a. when a schedule mix-up occurs
    b. when the client disagrees with you
    c. when you are certain that the client is wrong
    d. never ____

15. What is a goal of the "assess" consultation step?
    a. determine your client's objectives
    b. discuss topics like home care
    c. discus products the client uses
    d. Fitzpatrick typing

16. What is body language?
    a. the set of scientific terms used for describing the body
    b. any terminology the client uses to describe his or her body
    c. verbal communication such as describing which area will be treated
    d. nonverbal communication such as crossing your arms and frowning

17. What is an example of sensitivity?
    a. telling a brand-new client she looks terrible but you can help
    b. choosing your words carefully
    c. reminding a co-worker that her hairstyle is out of fashion
    d. swearing in the workplace

18. What is true of listening?
    a. it accomplishes less than talking
    b. listening too closely makes most people uncomfortable
    c. too much listening means not enough talking
    d. it is the best relationship builder

19. According to the golden rules of human relations, what does every action bring?
    a. reaction   c. verbal response
    b. inaction   d. physical response

20. What is also known as a client questionnaire?
    a. beauty review   c. consent form
    b. intake form   d. color chart

21. What is a primary ingredient for success in any career?
    a. ability to express your ideas in a forceful manner
    b. ability to manipulate other people into doing what you want
    c. ability to manipulate people into believing what you believe
    d. ability to express your ideas in a professional manner

22. Why is customer service important in esthetics?
    a. it is central to success
    b. treating customers well is the only way to make them tip generously
    c. treating customers well is the only way to get promoted
    d. it is not important in esthetics

23. What can you do when you begin with a firm understanding of yourself?
    a. manipulate others
    b. persuade others
    c. impress others
    d. understand others _____

24. What is an attitude adjustment?
    a. modification when emotions are interfering with work
    b. scolding you give to a client who is being annoying
    c. disciplinary action a manager makes to a misbehaving employee
    d. relaxation you feel when you leave work at the end of the day _____

25. What is constructive criticism?
    a. observations you offer about why a client does not look good
    b. comments you make about how other estheticians do their jobs
    c. feedback you provide when your manager is not performing well
    d. guidance offered by supervisors to improve your job performance _____

26. What do you exercise when you ensure that client information is kept private?
    a. sensitivity
    b. confidentiality
    c. duplicity
    d. courtesy _____

27. What do you exercise by not "picking a side" in a conflict?
    a. confidentiality
    b. hypocrisy
    c. neutrality
    d. sensitivity _____

28. What is a goal of the "maintenance" consultation step?
    a. discuss home care
    b. Fitzpatrick typing
    c. O'Malley typing
    d. discuss products the client uses _____

29. What type of cue is a smile?
    a. negative verbal
    b. positive verbal
    c. negative nonverbal
    d. positive nonverbal _____

30. What type of cue are hand gestures that are used to scold or embarrass?
    a. negative verbal
    b. positive verbal
    c. negative nonverbal
    d. positive nonverbal _____

31. What is a goal of the "preference" consultation step?
    a. discuss products the client uses
    b. discuss home care
    c. recommend new products
    d. determine skin type
    _____

32. What is our emotional state when we feel secure?
    a. sad, nervous, and unsure
    b. happy, calm, and confident
    c. arrogant, cocky, and obnoxious
    d. bored, calm, and tired
    _____

33. What should you remember when someone seems insensitive?
    a. people are genetically predetermined to be sensitive or insensitive
    b. you probably caused their insensitivity with your actions
    c. you probably caused their insensitivity with your words
    d. at this particular time, the person is feeling insecure
    _____

34. What should you avoid doing when confronted with bad behavior?
    a. responding calmly
    b. counting to 10 before speaking
    c. considering the other person's mood
    d. overreacting
    _____

35. What are you able to do when you believe in yourself?
    a. win every argument because you have confidence
    b. trust your judgment and uphold your own values
    c. convince clients to buy anything since you're so persuasive
    d. change your own values whenever it is convenient to do so
    _____

36. Why should you be attentive with all clients to learn what they want?
    a. in order to sell them products
    b. all clients are different
    c. in order to earn generous tips
    d. all clients want the same things
    _____

37. What is the act of successfully sharing information between people?
    a. networking   c. gossiping
    b. espionage   d. communication
    _____

38. What should happen *before* beginning any part of the service?
    a. Fitzpatrick typing   c. client consultation
    b. product recommendation d. aromatherapy
    _____

39. Why should client consultations be performed with as much privacy as possible?
    a. because they are embarrassing
    b. to avoid breaches of confidentiality
    c. so other estheticians cannot steal your clients
    d. so the manager won't hear if you make mistakes ____

40. When does the "review" step occur in the consultation process?
    a. at the beginning   c. whenever is convenient
    b. somewhere in the middle   d. at the end ____

41. When does the "repeat" step occur in the consultation process?
    a. at the end   c. somewhere in the middle
    b. whenever is convenient   d. at the beginning ____

42. What is reflective listening?
    a. repeating sales pitches taught to you by manufacturer's representatives
    b. watching the client's face in the mirror while she is speaking
    c. closing your eyes while someone speaks so you listen more closely
    d. repeating, in your own words, what you think the client has said ____

43. Why is the "repeat" step the most critical of the consultation process?
    a. clients don't pay attention until the end of the consultation
    b. it ultimately determines the service(s) you will perform
    c. everything you say in this step is considered a legal obligation
    d. your manager will be present for this step of the consultation ____

44. What is proven by the fact that human beings desire to interact with other people when they feel secure?
    a. everyone is basically lonely
    b. insecure people don't have friends
    c. people choose when to feel secure or insecure
    d. human beings are social animals ____

45. When should you ask for help, according to the golden rules of human relations?
    a. when you feel lazy
    b. when you feel overwhelmed
    c. when you feel lonely
    d. when you dislike your client ____

Part 2: General Sciences

CHAPTER 5—INFECTION CONTROL: PRINCIPLES AND PRACTICES

1. What term refers to the ability to produce an effect?
   a. efficacy
   b. disinfection
   c. motility
   d. sterilization   ____

2. What term indicates that a product is capable of destroying bacteria?
   a. bacteriphobic
   b. bacterial
   c. probacterial
   d. bactericidal   ____

3. What term refers to a resistance to disease that is partly inherited and partly developed through healthy living?
   a. natural immunity
   b. physical immunity
   c. acquired immunity
   d. healthy immunity   ____

4. What is scabies?
   a. bloodborne virus that causes disease
   b. type of fungus that affects plants or grows on inanimate objects
   c. superficial fungal infection that commonly affects the skin
   d. contagious disease caused by the itch mite   ____

5. What does the term *porous* mean?
   a. made or constructed of a material that does not have openings
   b. made or constructed of a material that has openings
   c. susceptible to disease
   d. immune to a disease   ____

6. What are bacilli?
   a. round-shaped bacteria
   b. spherical bacteria that grow in pairs
   c. spiral or corkscrew-shaped bacteria
   d. short, rod-shaped bacteria   ____

7. What are staphylococci?
   a. pus-forming bacterial that grow in clusters like a bunch of grapes
   b. spiral- or corkscrew-shaped bacteria that cause diseases such as syphilis
   c. microscopic plant parasites, including molds and mildews
   d. slender, hair-like extensions used by parasites for locomotion   ____

8. What are flagella?
   a. microscopic plant parasites, including molds and mildews
   b. pus-forming bacteria that grow in clusters like a bunch of grapes
   c. slender, hair-like extensions used by parasites for locomotion
   d. spiral- or corkscrew-shaped bacteria that cause diseases
      such as syphilis   _____

9. What is a microscopic germ that normally exists in tap water in
   small numbers?
   a. diplococci
   b. mycobacterium fortuitum
   c. human immunodeficiency virus
   d. mildew   _____

10. What is methicillin-resistant staphylococcus aureus?
    a. superficial fungal infection that commonly affects the skin
    b. microscopic germ that normally exists in tap water
    c. pus-forming bacteria that grow in clusters like bunches of
       grapes
    d. type of infectious bacteria that is highly resistant to antibiotics   _____

11. What is a responsibility of the Environmental Protection Agency
    (EPA)?
    a. testing and approving drugs sold and used in the
       United States
    b. overseeing all agricultural practices of U.S. farmers
    c. supervising employee safety in U.S. workplaces
    d. registering all types of disinfectants sold and used in
       the United States   _____

12. When happened in 1985 that triggered the creation of Universal
    Precautions?
    a. bird flu pandemic
    b. AIDS public health crisis
    c. hepatitis pandemic
    d. evidence of the return of the bubonic plague   _____

13. What is a responsibility of the Centers for Disease Control and
    Prevention (CDC)?
    a. reviewing and approving pharmaceutical products
    b. testing and licensing medical professionals
    c. testing and approving preparation techniques for food products
    d. studying diseases and providing guidance to prevent their spread   _____

14. What set of practices replaced Universal Precautions in 1996?
    a. Standard Precautions   c. Standard Procedures
    b. Global Precautions   d. Global Procedures   ____

15. When should an adhesive bandage be used?
    a. after breaking a pimple
    b. in response to an exposure incident
    c. prior to a dermabrasion treatment
    d. during tweezing to aid hair removal   ____

16. What is true of cardiopulmonary resuscitation (CPR)?
    a. it should only be performed by licensed medical professionals
    b. it is a basic element of first aid every esthetician should know
    c. only the salon manager is authorized to perform CPR
    d. you should only perform CPR if a client gives you verbal
       permission   ____

17. When should you call emergency medical technicians (EMTs)?
    a. only if it appears that someone in the salon is in moral danger
    b. as soon as possible after any significant accident has occurred
    c. only after you have exhausted your knowledge of first-aid
       techniques
    d. after the worst results of an accident have been addressed ____

18. How many levels of burns are there?
    a. three   c. six
    b. four   d. eight   ____

19. What is a fluid created by infection?
    a. mold   c. lymph
    b. mildew   d. pus   ____

20. What is the term for illness related to conditions associated with
    employment?
    a. employment disorder   c. occupational disorder
    b. employment disease   d. occupational disease   ____

21. What part of the body does tinea pedis affect?
    a. hands   c. knees
    b. elbows   d. feet   ____

22. What disease is caused by bacteria transmitted through coughing
    or sneezing?
    a. tuberculosis   c. hepatitis
    b. AIDS   d. diabetes   ____

23. What is the term for any organism of microscopic or submicroscopic size?
    a. miniorganism
    c. microorganism
    b. suborganism
    d. quasiorganism _____

24. What is the body fluid or secretion to which Standard Precautions do **NOT** apply?
    a. blood
    c. pus
    b. saliva
    d. sweat _____

25. When should you apply a mask, eyewear, or gown, according to Standard Precautions?
    a. whenever you come in contact with the human body
    b. if the splashing of body fluids is likely
    c. if the splashing of treatment products is likely
    d. whenever you come in contact with a pregnant client _____

26. What should you do **FIRST** when responding to an exposure incident?
    a. call an ambulance
    c. stop the bleeding
    b. disinfect your hands
    d. stop the service _____

27. When in the process of responding to an exposure incident should you recommend that the client see a physician if symptoms develop?
    a. at the beginning of the process
    b. in the middle of the process
    c. at the end of the process
    d. several times throughout the process _____

28. What term refers to disease-causing microorganisms carried in the body by blood?
    a. bloodstream invaders
    c. bloodborne invaders
    b. bloodstream pathogens
    d. bloodborne pathogens _____

29. What is infection control?
    a. wearing protective gear at all times in the salon
    b. methods used to eliminate or reduce transmission of infectious organisms
    c. methods that ensure absolutely no infections organisms enter the salon
    d. step-by-step instructions for performing medical aesthetic treatments _____

30. What term refers to the process for properly handling sterilized and disinfected equipment and supplies to reduce contamination?
   a. infection control
   b. infection procedures
   c. aseptic control
   d. aseptic procedures

   ____

31. What is the difference between rules and laws?
   a. laws are more specific than rules
   b. you are not expected to obey rules
   c. each salon makes up its own rules
   d. rules are more specific than laws

   ____

32. Which organization regulates and enforces safety standards to protect employees at work?
   a. Food and Drug Administration (FDA)
   b. United States Department of Agriculture (USDA)
   c. Centers for Disease Control and Prevention (CDC)
   d. Occupational Safety and Health Administration (OSHA)

   ____

33. What can you find on Material Safety Data Sheets (MSDSs)?
   a. lists of companies that sell the specified product
   b. information about possible hazards and safe use of products
   c. product pricing information
   d. comparison charts describing efficacy of similar products

   ____

34. What must every employee in the salon do after reading each MSDS that comes into the salon?
   a. verify having read the MSDS
   b. memorize the entire MSDS
   c. write a report on the MSDS
   d. copy the MSDS by hand

   ____

35. What part of the body is **MOST** often affected by folliculitis?
   a. eyebrows
   b. bridge of the nose
   c. armpits
   d. bearded areas of the face

   ____

36. What term indicates that a product is capable of destroying viruses?
   a. antibacterial
   b. neutroviral
   c. virucidal
   d. viruphobic

   ____

37. What term indicates that a person shows no signs or symptoms of infection?
   a. asymptomatic
   b. antisymptomatic
   c. symptomatic
   d. nonsymptomatic

   ____

38. What term refers to a reaction caused by extreme sensitivity to a normally harmless substance?
   a. analogy
   b. infection
   c. allergy
   d. contagion
   _____

39. What is the term for the number of viable organisms in or on an object or surface?
   a. bioload
   b. bioburden
   c. viable load
   d. viable burden
   _____

40. What is true of touching?
   a. touching is harmless since infection cannot be spread through touching
   b. it is rare for infection to be spread through touching
   c. every time you touch someone, you will get an infection
   d. touching is the most common method of spreading infection
   _____

41. What does the term *immunity* refer to?
   a. physical characteristics of people who are always sick
   b. ability of the body to easily absorb infection
   c. ability of the body to destroy and resist infection
   d. physical characteristics of people who are never sick
   _____

42. What term refers to the invasion of body tissues by disease-causing pathogens?
   a. inoculation
   b. allergy
   c. motility
   d. infection
   _____

43. What is the condition in which the body reacts to injury, irritation, or infection?
   a. inflammation
   b. immunity
   c. integrity
   d. incapacitation
   _____

44. What is sterilization?
   a. degree of cleansing acquired by rising with tap water
   b. process that completely destroys all microbial life
   c. process that destroys most, but not all, microorganisms on a surface
   d. degree of cleansing acquired by washing one's hands
   _____

45. What is a type of fungus that affects plants or grows on inanimate objects?
   a. pus
   b. mildew
   c. lymph
   d. spirilla
   _____

46. What is true of fourth-degree burns?
    a. they are not very serious
    b. they the most common type of burn
    c. they always require medical attention
    d. they are always fatal   _____

47. What term refers to a parasitic particle that infects and resides in
    the cells of biological organisms?
    a. fungus   c. bacteria
    b. immunization   d. virus   _____

48. What term refers to various poisonous substances produced by
    some microorganisms?
    a. quats   c. phenols
    b. toxins   d. flagella   _____

49. What is the common term for tinea versicolor?
    a. migraine   c. athlete's foot
    b. sun spots   d. barber's itch   _____

50. What is a systemic disease?
    a. disease that affects only one particular body system
    b. disease that affects the body as a whole
    c. disease that affects only two particular body systems
    d. disease that systematically runs its course in 24 hours _____

CHAPTER 6—GENERAL ANATOMY AND PHYSIOLOGY

1. How much blood does the human body contain?
   a. one to three pints
   b. eight to 10 pints
   c. 12 to 14 pints
   d. 17 to 20 pints   ____

2. What is a nutritive fluid flowing through the circulatory system?
   a. lymph
   b. blood
   c. pus
   d. water   ____

3. What are platelets?
   a. blood components that contribute to the blood-clotting process
   b. a type of white blood cell
   c. a type of red blood cell
   d. dangerous bacteria found in the bloodstream   ____

4. What is another term for white blood cells?
   a. capillaries
   b. leukocytes
   c. arterioles
   d. venules   ____

5. What is the study of tiny structures found in living tissues?
   a. anatomy
   b. physiology
   c. histology
   d. osteology   ____

6. What is one reason estheticians should study body systems, organs, and tissues?
   a. to obtain the medical license needed to become an esthetician
   b. to perform emergency surgery in the salon
   c. to prescribe medications for clients with skin disorders
   d. to understand the effect services have on the body   ____

7. What is protoplasm?
   a. foundation of all chemical beauty products
   b. substance of which the cells of all living things are composed
   c. toxic substance found in the bodies of people with diseases
   d. yellowish fluid that oozes from open sores   ____

8. What is the process of cell reproduction called?
   a. anagen
   b. catagen
   c. mitosis
   d. metastasization   ____

9. What is the sternum?
   a. flat bone that forms the ventral support of the ribs
   b. uppermost bone of the skull
   c. longest bone in the foot
   d. collarbone   _____

10. What part of the hand is supplied by the radical nerve and its
    branches?
    a. palm   c. pinky and ring fingers
    b. back   d. middle and index fingers   _____

11. What is the fluid part of the blood and lymph that carries food
    and secretions to the cells and carbon dioxide from the cells?
    a. pus   c. plasma
    b. lymph   d. sebum   _____

12. What is true of the origin part of a muscle?
    a. it is not attached to the skeleton
    b. it disappears after puberty
    c. it moves frequently
    d. it is attached to the skeleton   _____

13. What are structures composed of specialized tissues and
    performing specific functions?
    a. cells   c. body systems
    b. organs   d. bodies   _____

14. Why does the parathyroid gland regulate blood calcium and
    phosphorous levels?
    a. so the endocrine and muscular systems can function properly
    b. so the nervous and muscular systems can function properly
    c. so the nervous and circulatory systems can function properly
    d. so the endocrine and circulatory systems can function properly _____

15. What is true of the pituitary gland?
    a. it is the most complex organ of the endocrine system
    b. it is the most complex organ of the integumentary system
    c. it has no effect on the physiological processes of the body
    d. it affects very few of the body's physiological processes   _____

16. What organ in the endocrine system secretes enzyme-producing
    cells that are responsible for digesting carbohydrates, proteins,
    and fats?
    a. pancreas   c. liver
    b. kidney   d. stomach   _____

17. What are the secretions that the endocrine glands release directly into the bloodstream and that influence the welfare of the entire body?
    a. red blood cells
    b. white blood cells
    c. endorphins
    d. hormones
    _____

18. What is the primary function of the respiratory system?
    a. digestion
    b. blood circulation
    c. reproduction
    d. breathing
    _____

19. What is the primary function of the lymphatic/immune system?
    a. protecting the body from disease
    b. providing the body's outer shell
    c. facilitating reproduction
    d. facilitating respiration
    _____

20. What is the primary function of the skeletal system?
    a. providing the exterior protective covering of the body
    b. circulating blood to the bones and to muscles attached to bones
    c. circulating oxygen to the bones and to muscles attached to bones
    d. providing the physical foundation of the body
    _____

21. What is osteology?
    a. study of the muscles
    b. study of the bones
    c. study of the organs
    d. study of the blood
    _____

22. What is a term that means *bone* and is used as a prefix in many medical terms?
    a. os
    b. es
    c. as
    d. is
    _____

23. What is the primary function of the circulatory system?
    a. promoting sebum production
    b. providing a path for waste products to move out of the body
    c. providing carbon dioxide to all cells of the body
    d. moving blood through the body
    _____

24. What is covered, shaped, and supported by the muscular system?
    a. integumentary system
    b. skeletal tissue
    c. vital organs
    d. secondary organs
    _____

25. What body system is responsible for changing food into nutrients and waste?
    a. endocrine
    b. integumentary
    c. excretory
    d. digestive
    _____

26. What is the primary function of the excretory system?
    a. purifying the body by elimination of waste matter
    b. converting food into nutrients and waste
    c. circulating blood and lymph throughout the body
    d. circulating nitrogen and oxygen throughout the body   _____

27. What is the primary function of the reproductive system?
    a. discharging waste from the body
    b. perpetuating the human race
    c. maintaining erogenous zones
    d. feeding nutrients into the body   _____

28. What is the body system that controls and coordinates all other body systems?
    a. endocrine   c. integumentary
    b. reproductive   d. nervous   _____

29. What is a connection between two or more bones of the skeleton?
    a. joint   c. origin
    b. ligament   d. insertion   _____

30. What body system serves as a protective covering for the body?
    a. endocrine   c. nervous
    b. skeletal   d. integumentary   _____

31. What is a collection of similar cells that perform a particular function?
    a. lymph   c. body system
    b. sebum   d. tissue   _____

32. What are valves?
    a. structures that close a passage or permit flow in one direction only
    b. exterior openings on the body such as aural canals, nostrils, and pores
    c. junctures in the digestive system where food is halted and processed
    d. junctures in the excretory system where waste is halted and processed   _____

33. Where in the skull is the occipital bone located?
    a. front   c. left side
    b. back   d. right side   _____

34. How many identical daughter cells are formed when a cell divides during mitosis?
    a. two
    b. four
    c. six
    d. eight
    ____

35. What are the two phases of metabolism?
    a. anabolism and catabolism
    b. botulism and embolism
    c. internal and external
    d. primary and secondary
    ____

36. What is the metabolic process of building up larger molecules from smaller ones?
    a. premetabolism
    b. postmetabolism
    c. anabolism
    d. catabolism
    ____

37. When, during metabolism, are complex compounds within the cells broken down into smaller ones?
    a. anabolism
    b. catabolism
    c. primary metabolism
    d. secondary metabolism
    ____

38. What body system affects the growth, development, sexual activities, and health of the body?
    a. circulatory
    b. integumentary
    c. nervous
    d. endocrine
    ____

39. Where in the body does the spinal cord originate?
    a. top of the skull
    b. base of the neck
    c. brain
    d. heart
    ____

40. What are glands?
    a. sexual organs required for reproduction
    b. specialized organs that remove and convert elements from the blood
    c. chambers of the heart required for circulation
    d. groups of cells in the skin responsible for perspiration
    ____

41. What are lymph nodes?
    a. gland-like structures found inside the lymphatic vessels
    b. components of lymph that flow through lymphatic vessels
    c. dedicated muscles that power the lymphatic vessels
    d. tubes that take lymph to and from lymphatic vessels
    ____

42. What are two physical characteristics of lymph?
    a. thick and sticky
    b. red and spongy
    c. yellow and gelatinous
    d. colorless and watery
    ____

43. What binds tissues of the body together?
    a. anatomical binders   c. adhesive tissue
    b. physiological binders   d. connective tissue   _____

44. What type of tissue provides a protective covering on body surfaces?
    a. endocrine   c. nerve
    b. epithelial   d. border   _____

45. What carries messages to and from the brain and controls and coordinates all body functions?
    a. epithelial tissue   c. nerve tissue
    b. cardiac tissue   d. supervisory tissue   _____

46. What organ circulates the blood?
    a. brain   c. liver
    b. heart   d. kidney   _____

47. What do the kidneys do?
    a. pump nitrogen into the blood
    b. pump oxygen into the blood
    c. convert food to nutrients
    d. excrete water and waste products   _____

48. What is the name of the two bones that form the bridge of the nose?
    a. occipital   c. nasal
    b. cranial   d. dorsal   _____

49. What is the largest and strongest bone in the face?
    a. lacrimal   c. mandible
    b. vomer   d. turbinal   _____

50. What is formed by the 12 pairs of bones in the ribs?
    a. sternum   c. epiglottis
    b. thorax   d. abdomen   _____

51. What serves as the protective framework for the heart, lungs, and other internal organs?
    a. thorax   c. abdomen
    b. sternum   d. torso   _____

52. What are small vessels that connect capillaries to veins?
    a. granules   c. ampules
    b. papules   d. venules   _____

53. What term refers to thin-walled blood vessels that are less elastic than arteries?
    a. venules
    b. veins
    c. vesicles
    d. ventricles
    _____

54. What gland controls how quickly the body burns energy and makes proteins?
    a. adrenal
    b. pineal
    c. pituitary
    d. thyroid
    _____

55. What is **NOT** true about the brain?
    a. it is where thoughts are formed
    b. it is the largest organ of the body
    c. it controls the body
    d. it is protected by the cranium
    _____

56. What supplies oxygen to the blood?
    a. brain
    b. heart
    c. lungs
    d. kidneys
    _____

57. What is the function of the liver?
    a. removing waste created by digestion
    b. circulating lymph through the body
    c. adding oxygen to the blood
    d. removing oxygen from the blood
    _____

58. What organ aids the intestines in the digestion of food?
    a. kidney
    b. liver
    c. stomach
    d. pancreas
    _____

59. What is defecation?
    a. circulating water through the body
    b. breaking food down into nutrients
    c. absorbing nutrients into the body
    d. eliminating waste from the body
    _____

60. What is the term for taking food into the body?
    a. ingestion
    b. digestion
    c. indigestion
    d. regurgitation
    _____

CHAPTER 7—BASICS OF CHEMISTRY

1. What has physical properties that we can see, smell, taste, and touch?
    a. radiation
    b. matter
    c. energy
    d. electricity
    _____

2. What causes oxidation?
    a. addition of oxygen or the loss of hydrogen
    b. addition of hydrogen or the loss of oxygen
    c. addition of both oxygen and hydrogen
    d. loss of both oxygen and hydrogen
    _____

3. What is an ion?
    a. atom or molecule that carries an electrical charge
    b. atom or molecule without an electrical charge
    c. dust particle left over after the ionization process
    d. spark discharged during the ionization process
    _____

4. What is an atom with a positive electrical charge?
    a. neutron
    b. anion
    c. cation
    d. molecule
    _____

5. What is an ion with a negative charge?
    a. anion
    b. cation
    c. molecule
    d. neutron
    _____

6. What does the term *miscible* mean?
    a. incapable of being mixed
    b. capable of being mixed
    c. incapable of being ionized
    d. capable of being ionized
    _____

7. What is united with the aid of an emulsifier to create an emulsion?
    a. two or more miscible substances
    b. two or more immiscible substances
    c. a reduction and a solution
    d. a surfactant and a liquid
    _____

8. What is a solution?
    a. stable mixture of an emulsion and a reduction
    b. unstable mixture of an emulsion and a reduction
    c. uniform mixture of two or more mutually immiscible substances
    d. uniform mixture of two or more mutually miscible substances
    _____

9. What is air?
   a. shell of radiation surrounding Earth
   b. gaseous mixture that makes up the Earth's atmosphere
   c. common name for the chemical that makes the sky appear blue
   d. water vapor that forms clouds ____

10. What is true of liquid?
   a. it is matter with fixed volume and definite shape
   b. it is matter with no fixed volume and no definite shape
   c. it is matter with fixed volume but no definite shape
   d. it is matter with no fixed volume but definite shape ____

11. What is **NOT** true of atoms?
   a. all matter is composed of atoms
   b. they are small particles of elements
   c. all atoms are identical
   d. atoms consist of smaller particles ____

12. What is true of oxygen?
   a. it is the most abundant element on Earth
   b. it is the least abundant element on Earth
   c. it should not be ingested because it is poisonous to humans
   d. contrary to popular belief, there is no oxygen in the air ____

13. What is true of water?
   a. it is the most abundant of all substances on Earth
   b. it is a relatively scarce substance
   c. water comprises a very small portion of the human body
   d. the human body is made entirely of water ____

14. What is true of elements?
   a. there are only five basic elements in the universe
   b. in chemistry, the main elements are sunshine, clouds, rain, and snow
   c. elements are the most complex form of matter
   d. elements are the simplest form of matter ____

15. What is light a form of?
   a. energy   c. gas
   b. matter   d. liquid ____

16. What is true of each of the approximately 90 naturally occurring elements?
    a. though chemical properties vary, all have the same physical properties
    b. though physical properties vary, all have the same chemical properties
    c. all share the same physical and chemical properties
    d. each has its own distinctive physical and chemical properties _____

17. What term refers to molecules that contain two or more atoms of the same element?
    a. atomic molecules
    b. chemical molecules
    c. radiological molecules
    d. elemental molecules _____

18. What businesses primarily use oil-in-water emulsions?
    a. auto repair shops
    b. bakeries
    c. salons and spas
    d. fast-food restaurants _____

19. What is true of moisturizer?
    a. it is an oil-in-water emulsion
    b. it is a water-in-oil emulsion
    c. it is an oil-in-water reduction
    d. it is a water-in-oil reduction _____

20. What is a difference between water-in-oil (W/O) emulsions and oil-in-water (O/W) emulsions?
    a. O/W emulsions are greasier
    b. W/O emulsions are greasier
    c. O/W emulsions are not easily rinsed away with water
    d. W/O emulsions are easily rinsed away with water _____

21. What are most skin care products?
    a. reductions of oil and water
    b. emulsions of oil and water
    c. solutions of oil and water
    d. suspensions of oil and water _____

22. What term means "water-loving"?
    a. hydrocentric
    b. hydroactive
    c. hydrophobic
    d. hydrophilic _____

23. What term means "oil-loving"?
    a. lipophilic
    b. lipocentric
    c. lipoactive
    d. lipophobic _____

24. How much of the air is made up of nitrogen?
    a. one-quarter   c. two-thirds
    b. three-eighths   d. four-fifths   ____

25. What is the science that deals with the composition, structure, and properties of matter and how matter changes under different conditions?
    a. physiology   c. biology
    b. ergonomics   d. chemistry   ____

26. What are the two branches of chemistry?
    a. alkaline and acidic   c. anagen and catagen
    b. organic and inorganic   d. artificial and natural ____

27. What element is absent from the compounds studied in inorganic chemistry?
    a. nitrogen   c. carbon
    b. oxygen   d. helium   ____

28. What is the study of substances that contain carbon?
    a. carbon chemistry   c. organic chemistry
    b. carbon dating   d. organic dating   ____

29. What element is found in all living things, whether they are plants or animals?
    a. zinc   c. radon
    b. helium   d. carbon   ____

30. What is any substance that is dissolved by a solvent to form a solution?
    a. suspension   c. solute
    b. matter   d. emulsion   ____

31. What do antioxidants prevent by neutralizing free radicals?
    a. radicalization   c. oxygenation
    b. oxidation   d. ionization   ____

32. What type of neutralization reaction forms water and salt?
    a. reduction-compound   c. acid-alkali
    b. atom-alkali   d. solution-compound   ____

33. What is the natural pH of the skin?
    a. 3.5   c. 7.0
    b. 5.5   d. 7.5   ____

34. What term refers to substances with a pH below 7.0?
    a. acids   c. bases
    b. alkalis   d. solutes   _____

35. What are substances with a pH above 7.0?
    a. acids   c. reductions
    b. alkalis   d. solutions   _____

36. What type of substance has a pH level of 7.0?
    a. alkaline   c. neutral
    b. acidic   d. toxic   _____

37. What are surfactants?
    a. chemical compounds made from a reduction and a solution
    b. chemical compounds made from a reduction and a
       suspension
    c. unstable mixtures of two or more immiscible substances
    d. stable mixtures of two or more immiscible substances   _____

38. What is reduction?
    a. loss of both oxygen and hydrogen
    b. addition of both oxygen and hydrogen
    c. loss of oxygen or the addition of hydrogen
    d. addition of oxygen or the loss of hydrogen   _____

39. What is the term that refers to matter in its three physical forms
    (liquid, solid, gas)?
    a. states of matter   c. appearances of matter
    b. physical properties   d. chemical properties   _____

40. How much of the Earth's surface, approximately, is water?
    a. 10 percent   c. 75 percent
    b. 25 percent   d. 100 percent   _____

CHAPTER 8—BASICS OF ELECTRICITY

1. What does the acronym LED stand for?
   a. light-emitting diode
   b. laser-emitting device
   c. light electrical device
   d. laser electrode dial
   _____

2. What measure is one-thousandth of an ampere?
   a. multiampere
   b. milliampere
   c. microampere
   d. macroampere
   _____

3. What term refers to currents used as electrical facial and scalp treatments?
   a. modems
   b. moderations
   c. modalities
   d. modes
   _____

4. What apparatus changes alternating current to direct current?
   a. charger
   b. actuator
   c. modifier
   d. rectifier
   _____

5. What describes Tesla high-frequency current?
   a. high rate of oscillation and a low rate of vibration
   b. high rate of oscillation and vibration
   c. low rate of oscillation and vibration
   d. low rate of oscillation and a high rate of vibration
   _____

6. What is a description of white light?
   a. complete absence of light of any color
   b. combination of all the visible rays of the spectrum
   c. combination of all the invisible rays of the spectrum
   d. combination of any two or more colors of visible light
   _____

7. What is yellow LED light used for?
   a. aiding in facial and scalp treatments
   b. detoxifying the skin
   c. reducing inflammation and swelling
   d. stimulating circulation
   _____

8. What is red LED light used for?
   a. stimulating circulation
   b. reducing inflammation and swelling
   c. detoxifying the skin
   d. aiding in facial and scalp treatments
   _____

9. What is green LED light used for?
   a. aiding in facial and scalp treatments
   b. reducing inflammation and swelling
   c. stimulating circulation
   d. detoxifying the skin   _____

10. What is the primary source of light used in facial and scalp treatments?
    a. visible light   c. natural light
    b. invisible light   d. artificial light   _____

11. What is a device in which UVA radiation is used?
    a. autoclave   c. hairdryer
    b. tanning bed   d. towel warner   _____

12. What is a term commonly used in reference to UVB radiation?
    a. tanning light   c. ozone light
    b. rainbow light   d. burning light   _____

13. What is true of UVC radiation?
    a. it is the least dangerous type of UV radiation
    b. it is the most dangerous type of UV radiation
    c. it is used in tanning beds
    d. it is often called the burning light   _____

14. What term refers to a color component within the skin such as blood or melanin?
    a. chromoform   c. chromakey
    b. chromophore   d. chromazyme   _____

15. How does red LED light affect cellular processes?
    a. decreases cellular processes
    b. increases cellular processes
    c. stops cellular processes completely
    d. interrupts cellular processes temporarily   _____

16. What is **NOT** a condition that intense pulsed light is used to treat?
    a. spider veins   c. albinism
    b. hyperpigmentation   d. excessive light   _____

17. What is wavelength?
    a. primary source of light used in facial and scalp treatments
    b. distance between two successive peaks of electromagnetic waves
    c. flow of electricity along a conductor
    d. color component of the skin found at different depths   _____

18. What does a watt measure?
    a. how much electric energy is used in one second
    b. how much electric energy is used in 10 seconds
    c. how much electric energy is used in one minute
    d. how much electric energy is used in 10 minutes   _____

19. What do volts measure?
    a. force pushing electrons forward through a conductor
    b. force moving protons backward through a conductor
    c. resistance keeping electrons from moving through a conductor
    d. resistance keeping protons from moving through a conductor   _____

20. What do ohms measure?
    a. force of electric current
    b. direction of electric current
    c. resistance of electric current
    d. absence of electric current   _____

21. What is the term for a rapid and interrupted current, flowing first
    in one direction and then in the opposite direction?
    a. direct current   c. advanced current
    b. alternating current   d. directional current   _____

22. What is the term for a constant, even-flowing current that travels
    in one direction only?
    a. steady current   c. even current
    b. direct current   d. alternating current   _____

23. What unit measures the amount of an electric current?
    a. ohm   c. volt
    b. watt   d. amp   _____

24. What type of LED light is used to treat acne?
    a. blue   c. yellow
    b. green   d. red   _____

25. What is the term for a negative electrode?
    a. diode   c. cathode
    b. anode   d. nullode   _____

26. What is the movement of particles around an atom that creates
    pure energy?
    a. fission   c. electricity
    b. fusion   d. magnetism   _____

27. What should you do on a regular basis?
    a. inspect electrical equipment
    b. submerge electrical equipment in water for cleaning purposes
    c. discard any electrical equipment that looks old-fashioned
    d. dismantle electrical equipment   _____

28. What is ionization?
    a. forcing acidic substances into deeper tissue using galvanic current
    b. introducing water-soluble products into the skin with electric current
    c. using galvanic current to create an alkaline chemical reaction
    d. the use of electrical devices for therapeutic benefits   _____

29. What is cataphoresis?
    a. forcing alkaline substances into deeper tissues using galvanic current
    b. withdrawing alkaline substances from the skin with microcurrent
    c. withdrawing acidic substances from the skin with microcurrent
    d. forcing acidic substances into deeper tissues using galvanic current   _____

30. What is anaphoresis?
    a. forcing liquids into tissues from the negative toward the positive pole
    b. forcing liquids into tissues from the positive toward the negative pole
    c. pulling liquids from tissues, from the negative toward the positive pole
    d. pulling liquids from tissues, from the positive toward the negative pole   _____

31. What is the other method for applying high-frequency current, besides indirect application?
    a. angular surface application
    b. angular superficial application
    c. indirect surface application
    d. indirect superficial application   _____

32. What percentage of natural sunlight does invisible infrared light comprise?
    a. 10   c. 60
    b. 30   d. 100   _____

33. What is a complete circuit?
    a. path of current from one conductor to the next
    b. path of current from the source through conductors and back
    c. path of current from the source to the first conductor
    d. path of current from the last conductor back to the source _____

34. What is the term for any substance that easily transmits electricity?
    a. transmitter   c. resister
    b. receiver   d. conductor _____

35. What is the device that prevents excessive current from passing through a circuit?
    a. switch   c. fuse
    b. outlet   d. ground _____

36. What completes a circuit and carries the current safely away?
    a. circuit breaker   c. fuse
    b. mainline   d. ground _____

37. What are invisible rays with long wavelengths?
    a. phantom light rays   c. translucent light rays
    b. infrared light rays   d. ethereal light rays _____

38. What is the term for a substance that does not easily transmit electricity?
    a. conductor   c. fuse
    b. insulator   d. circuit _____

39. What is the measurement for 1,000 watts?
    a. megawatt   c. kilowatt
    b. macrowatt   d. kerawatt _____

40. What is **NOT** a condition treated with light therapy?
    a. obesity   c. wrinkles
    b. capillaries   d. acne _____

CHAPTER 9—BASICS OF NUTRITION

1. What term refers to carbohydrates that contain three or more simple carbohydrate molecules?
   a. polysaccharides
   b. monosaccharides
   c. mucopolysaccharides
   d. disaccharides ____

2. What term refers to carbohydrate-lipid complexes that are also good water binders?
   a. disaccharides
   b. mucopolysaccharides
   c. monosaccharides
   d. polysaccharides ____

3. How are nonessential amino acids different from other amino acids?
   a. they are toxic to the human body
   b. they cannot be synthesized by the body and must be obtained from diet
   c. they can be synthesized by the body and need not be obtained from diet
   d. they are not among the 20 "common" amino acids ____

4. What is another name for alpha-linoleic acid, a type of "good" polyunsaturated fat that may decrease cardiovascular diseases?
   a. omega-3 fatty acids
   b. alpha-3 fatty acids
   c. omega-6 fatty acids
   d. alpha-6 fatty acids ____

5. What is the term for a thinning of the bones caused by the reabsorption of calcium into the bones?
   a. osteology
   b. osteoporosis
   c. osteohydrosis
   d. osteoculosis ____

6. What are proteins?
   a. inorganic materials
   b. macronutrients used to produce energy
   c. chains of amino acid molecules
   d. compounds that break down the basic chemical sugars ____

7. What is the commercial name for the vitamin-A derivative retinoic acid?
   a. Proactiv®
   b. Retin-A®
   c. Retino™
   d. Botox® ____

8. What is the vitamin from which tretinoin (used for collagen synthesis, hyperpigmentation, and acne) is derived?
   a. vitamin A
   b. vitamin C
   c. vitamin E
   d. vitamin K ____

9. What is one of the functions of the antioxidant vitamin A?
   a. facilitates the synthesis of factors necessary for blood coagulation
   b. aids in the functioning and repair of the skin cells
   c. essential for growth and development
   d. prevents collagen synthesis and is used to treat visible signs of aging _____

10. What is another name for vitamin C?
    a. ascorbic acid   c. sunshine vitamin
    b. retinol   d. tocopherol _____

11. What does adenosine triphosphate do?
    a. forms the building blocks of protein
    b. facilitates enzymatic reactions
    c. provides energy to cells and converts energy to carbon dioxide
    d. protects nerves and contributes to the structure of cells _____

12. What forms the building blocks of protein?
    a. bioflavonoids   c. adenosine triphosphate
    b. amino acids   d. carbohydrates _____

13. What is the term for clogging and hardening of the arteries?
    a. osteoporosis   c. hypoglycemia
    b. arteriosclerosis   d. arteriogylcemia _____

14. What food contains the greatest abundance of bioflavonoids?
    a. leafy greens   c. dairy products
    b. citrus fruits   d. whole grains _____

15. What are measures of heat units, used to measure food energy for the body?
    a. grams   c. pints
    b. calories   d. ounces _____

16. What are compounds that break down sugars and supply body energy?
    a. proteins   c. carbohydrates
    b. calories   d. enzymes _____

17. What term refers to sugars made up of two simple sugars, such as lactose and sucrose?
    a. bisaccharides   c. monosaccharides
    b. polysaccharides   d. disaccharides _____

18. What are catalysts that break down complex food molecules?
    a. carbohydrates   c. enzymes
    b. calories   d. proteins   _____

19. What type of vitamin is riboflavin?
    a. vitamin A   c. vitamin C
    b. vitamin B   d. vitamin D   _____

20. What mineral serves the function of forming and maintaining teeth and bones?
    a. calcium   c. iron
    b. iodine   d. copper   _____

21. What mineral is required for energy use, water balance, and molecular movement?
    a. magnesium   c. sodium
    b. calcium   d. potassium   _____

22. What mineral is required for energy release and protein synthesis?
    a. iron   c. magnesium
    b. calcium   d. potassium   _____

23. What mineral moves carbon dioxide, regulates water levels, and transports materials through cell membranes?
    a. potassium   c. iron
    b. sodium   d. calcium   _____

24. What is **NOT** an important reason for estheticians to develop and use good health habits?
    a. setting an example for clients
    b. having more energy for work
    c. seeking superficial approval
    d. trying to achieve personal balance   _____

25. How often should you exercise for about 30 minutes in order to maintain good health habits?
    a. twice a day   c. three times a week
    b. twice a week   d. five times a week   _____

26. What is true of water?
    a. you should only drink water after you exercise
    b. it can be refreshing but is not necessary for the body's health
    c. it is the one essential nutrient no person can live without
    d. you should only drink water when it is hot outside   _____

27. What are fats?
    a. chains of amino acid molecules
    b. macronutrients used to produce energy in the body
    c. inorganic materials required for many reactions of the cells
    d. organic acids that form protein
    _____

28. What has been added to a food product if it is labeled as fortified?
    a. flavor enhancer   c. one or more vitamins
    b. preservatives   d. sodium
    _____

29. What is glycosaminoglycan?
    a. water-binding substance between the fibers of the dermis
    b. substance that provides energy to the cells
    c. waxy substance in your body needed to produce hormones
    d. sugar made up of two simple sugars, such as lactose and sucrose
    _____

30. What is hypoglycemia?
    a. allergy to sugar
    b. inability to taste sugar
    c. condition in which blood sugar rises too high
    d. condition in which blood sugar drops too low
    _____

31. What is the common name for linoleic acid, which is used to make important hormones?
    a. omega-3   c. omega-9
    b. omega-6   d. omega-12
    _____

32. What is true of macronutrients?
    a. they are harmful to body systems and must be avoided
    b. they make up the largest part of the nutrition we take in
    c. they make up the smallest part of the nutrition we take in
    d. they offer nutrition without calories
    _____

33. What is true of micronutrients?
    a. they make up the largest part of the nutrition we take in
    b. they are high in fat and calories
    c. micronutrients have no calories or nutritional value
    d. they are harmful to body systems and must be avoided
    _____

34. What term refers to organic materials that are required for many reactions of the cells and the body?
    a. calories   c. carbohydrates
    b. enzymes   d. minerals
    _____

35. What term refers to carbohydrates made up of one basic sugar unit?
   a. unisaccharides
   c. polysaccharides
   b. disaccharides
   d. monosaccharides
   _____

36. What is a common name for vitamin D?
   a. sunshine vitamin
   c. ascorbic acid
   b. riboflavin
   d. skin vitamin
   _____

37. What is the scientific name for vitamin E?
   a. tocopherol
   c. retinol
   b. ascorbic acid
   d. linoleic acid
   _____

38. What body function is aided by vitamin K?
   a. healthy bone formation
   b. blood coagulation
   c. respiration of body organs
   d. red blood cell formation
   _____

39. What is a function of the United States Department of Agriculture (USDA)?
   a. overseeing financial transactions
   b. approving drugs for public use
   c. studying diseases
   d. regulating nutrition-related affairs
   _____

40. What is the governmental agency that issues the recommended nutritional guideline MyPlate?
   a. Centers for Disease Control and Prevention (CDC)
   b. Federal Trade Commission (FTC)
   c. United States Department of Agriculture (USDA)
   d. Food and Drug Administration (FDA)
   _____

41. What are recommended dietary allowances (RDAs)?
   a. government-issued measurements for amounts of foods we should eat
   b. industry-issued suggestions for amounts of food we should eat
   c. government-mandated requirements for amounts of food we should eat
   d. consumer-group recommendations for amounts of food we should eat
   _____

42. What type of vitamin is niacin?
    a. vitamin A   c. vitamin C
    b. vitamin B   d. vitamin D   _____

43. What mineral contributes to body tissue formation and gives strength to keratin?
    a. sulphur   c. selenium
    b. zinc   d. fluoride   _____

44. What mineral is commonly used in toothpaste because it contributes to bone and teeth formation?
    a. manganese   c. zinc
    b. fluoride   d. phosphorus   _____

Part 3: Skin Sciences

CHAPTER 10—PHYSIOLOGY AND HISTOLOGY OF THE SKIN

1. Why is UVB radiation also known as "burning rays"?
   a. UVB wavelengths cause burning of the skin as well as cancer
   b. UVB radiation burns paper upon direct exposure
   c. UVB radiation burns wood upon direct exposure
   d. UVB causes premature aging in skin _____

2. What is **NOT** an element of the skin's acid mantle?
   a. blood   c. lipids
   b. sebum   d. sweat _____

3. What causes injured skin to restore itself to its normal thickness?
   a. hyperproduction of cells   c. gentle massage
   b. daily exposure to the sun   d. Botox injections _____

4. What are the items in the dermis that respond to touch, pain, cold, heat, and pressure?
   a. sebaceous glands   c. fibrous tissues
   b. sensory nerve endings   d. pituitary glands _____

5. What are most abundant in the fingertips, as opposed to other parts of the body?
   a. red blood cells   c. lymph nodes
   b. white blood cells   d. sensory nerve fibers _____

6. What is the average internal temperature of the body in degrees Fahrenheit?
   a. 37   c. 98.6
   b. 96.8   d. 99.5 _____

7. Why does the body perspire?
   a. to protect us from overheating
   b. to protect us from freezing
   c. to protect us from dehydration
   d. to protect us from overhydration _____

8. What are follicles?
   a. sweat gland openings
   b. tubelike openings in the epidermis
   c. tubelike openings in the muscles
   d. ingrown hair shafts _____

9. What is **NOT** a compound in the body from which free radicals take electrons?
   a. sebum
   c. lipid
   b. protein
   d. DNA _____

10. What is glycation?
    a. fibrous, connective tissue made from protein
    b. a white blood cell that has enzymes to digest and kill bacteria
    c. the binding of a protein molecule to a glucose molecule
    d. a chronic condition that appears primarily in the cheeks _____

11. What are hair papillae?
    a. ingrown hairs
    b. cone-shaped elevations at the base of the follicle
    c. shaved hairs
    d. membranes of ridges and grooves that attach to the epidermis _____

12. Where in the body is hyaluronic acid found?
    a. hair
    c. kidney
    b. skin
    d. liver _____

13. What is hydrolipidic film?
    a. salt-water balance that damages the skin's surface
    b. oil-water balance that damages the skin's surface
    c. salt-water balance that protects the skin's surface
    d. oil-water balance that protects the skin's surface _____

14. What is a fiber protein found in skin, hair, and nails?
    a. keratin
    c. lymph
    b. keloid
    d. sebum _____

15. What is the acid mantle?
    a. deposit left on the skin after the use of an acidic product
    b. protective layer of lipids and secretions on the skin's surface
    c. reservoir of digestive juices located in the stomach
    d. deposit left on the skin after the use of an alkaline product _____

16. Where in the body are the coiled structures known as apocrine glands found?
    a. mouth and nostrils
    b. underarm and genital areas
    c. eyes and ears
    d. lower back and inner knees _____

17. What is the result of the contraction of the arrector pili muscle?
    a. penile erection   c. gaseous discharge
    b. excessive sweating   d. goose bumps   ____

18. What does the skin's barrier function protect us from, in addition
    to irritation?
    a. excessive hair loss   c. hyperpigmentation
    b. hypopigmentation   d. intercellular water loss   ____

19. What are ceramides?
    a. glycolipid materials   c. neurolipid materials
    b. hydrolipid materials   d. psycholipid materials   ____

20. What is collagen?
    a. hardened keratinocyte
    b. fibrous tissue made from protein
    c. hydrating fluid found in the skin
    d. pigment-carrying granule   ____

21. What are corneocytes?
    a. open comedones   c. closed comedones
    b. hardened kertatinocytes   d. softened keratinocytes   ____

22. What are membranes of ridges and grooves that attach to the
    epidermis?
    a. follicular papillae   c. epidermal papillae
    b. dermal papillae   d. hair papillae   ____

23. Where in the face does the chronic condition rosacea primarily
    appear?
    a. forehead and chin   c. jawline and ears
    b. ears and eyelids   d. cheeks and nose   ____

24. What protects the surface of the skin?
    a. hair papillae   c. pituitary glands
    b. sebaceous glands   d. dermal papillae   ____

25. What are guard cells of the immune system that sense
    unrecognized foreign invaders, such as bacteria?
    a. stratum germinativum
    b. stratum lucidum
    c. integumentary production cells
    d. Langerhans immune cells   ____

26. What is oil that provides protection for the epidermis from external factors and that lubricates both the skin and hair?
    a. lymph
    b. pus
    c. blood
    d. sebum
    ____

27. What is the common name for the stratum corneum?
    a. horny layer
    b. spiny layer
    c. granular layer
    d. clear layer
    ____

28. What is true of the stratum corneum?
    a. it is made of hardened sebum
    b. it is the outermost layer of the skin
    c. it is the innermost layer of the skin
    d. it is devoid of corneocytes
    ____

29. What is the common name of the stratum germiniativum?
    a. spiny layer
    b. basal layer
    c. horny layer
    d. clear layer
    ____

30. Where in the skin is the stratum germinativum located?
    a. below the papillary layer of the dermis
    b. below the hypodermis
    c. above the epidermis
    d. above the papillary layer of the dermis
    ____

31. What is the common name of the stratum granulosum?
    a. clear layer
    b. granular layer
    c. basal layer
    d. spiny layer
    ____

32. What forms the cells in the stratum granulosum that resemble granules?
    a. collagen
    b. keratin
    c. elastin
    d. melanin
    ____

33. What is the common name for the stratum corneum?
    a. horny layer
    b. clear layer
    c. basal layer
    d. spiny layer
    ____

34. What is another name for the subcutaneous layer of the skin?
    a. epidermis
    b. dermis
    c. hypodermis
    d. subdermis
    ____

35. What part of the skin provides a protective cushion and energy storage for the body?
    a. epidermis
    b. subcutaneous layer
    c. dermis
    d. barrier function
    ____

36. What is another name for subcutis tissue?
    a. acidic tissue   c. adipose tissue
    b. alkaline tissue   d. arrector tissue   _____

37. What are the glands that excrete perspiration, regulate body temperature, and detoxify the body?
    a. sudoriferous   c. hyperthyroid
    b. thyroid   d. pituitary   _____

38. What cells identify molecules that have foreign peptides, and help to regulate immune response?
    a. A-cells   c. T-cells
    b. D-cells   d. X-cells   _____

39. What causes telangiectasia?
    a. capillary damage   c. aging
    b. follicle damage   d. poor nutrition   _____

40. What causes transepidermal water loss?
    a. perspiration   c. salivation
    b. evaporation   d. secretion   _____

41. What is a common term for UVA radiation?
    a. aging rays   c. tanning rays
    b. burning rays   d. brightening rays   _____

42. What is the dermis?
    a. innermost layer of the skin
    b. outermost layer of the skin
    c. support layer above the epidermis
    d. support layer below the epidermis   _____

43. What function do desmosomes perform?
    a. assist in keeping cells apart   c. fight inflammation
    b. assist in holding cells together d. fight infection   _____

44. What are eccrine glands?
    a. tastebuds   c. salivary glands
    b. goosebumps   d. sweat glands   _____

45. What protein fiber is found in the dermis and gives skin its flexibility and firmness?
    a. collagen   c. keratin
    b. melanin   d. elastin   _____

46. What hormone stimulates cells to reproduce and heal?
    a. dermal stimulant factor (DSF)
    b. epidermal growth factor (EGF)
    c. integumentary regulatory factor (IRF)
    d. integumentary manufacturing factor (IMF)   _____

47. What is true of the epidermis?
    a. it is the outermost layer of the skin
    b. it is the innermost layer of the skin
    c. it is below the dermis
    d. it is below the subcutaneous layer   _____

48. What performs the function of stimulating cells, collagen, and
    amino acids that form proteins?
    a. epidermablasts   c. elastiblasts
    b. dermablasts   d. fibroblasts   _____

49. What term do clients commonly use when referring to follicles?
    a. blotches   c. pimples
    b. pores   d. rashes   _____

50. What comprises about 50 to 70 percent of the skin?
    a. lymph   c. oil
    b. water   d. pus   _____

51. What causes the body to produce its own vitamin D?
    a. drinking orange juice   c. drinking a liter of water
    b. exposure to the sun   d. exposure to heat   _____

52. What is **NOT** one of the six primary functions of the skin?
    a. heat regulation   c. absorption
    b. sensation   d. reflection   _____

53. What function does the enzyme tyrosinase perform?
    a. helps to regulate the body's internal temperature
    b. stimulates melanocytes and thus produces melanin
    c. triggers hyperproduction of cells and blood clotting
    d. helps to regulate the body's external temperature   _____

54. What is the other type of melanin the body produces, besides
    eumelanin?
    a. pheomelanin   c. pseudomelanin
    b. photomelanin   d. protomelanin   _____

55. How many times thicker than the epidermis is the dermis, approximately?
    a. 25
    b. 50
    c. 75
    d. 100 _____

56. When do free radicals produce more free radicals?
    a. before causing oxidation reactions
    b. while causing oxidation reactions
    c. only when exposed to hydrogen
    d. only when exposed to carbon _____

57. What causes skin cells' built-in antioxidants to lose their ability to protect cells?
    a. sun exposure
    b. sun deprivation
    c. excessive moisture
    d. excessive heat _____

58. What is true of sun exposure?
    a. all skin types benefit from extensive exposure to the sun
    b. of all factors, it has the least impact on how our skin ages
    c. of all factors, it has the greatest impact on how our skin ages
    d. several hours of sun exposure every day is recommended for the skin _____

59. What are keratinocytes?
    a. dermal cells composed of keratin, lipids, and other proteins
    b. epidermal cells composed of keratin, lipids, and other proteins
    c. dangerous bacteria that target and destroy keratin the body
    d. products that are unsafe to use because they deplete keratin _____

60. Where in the skin are lymph vessels located?
    a. dermis
    b. epidermis
    c. subcutaneous layer
    d. hypodermis _____

61. What protein determines hair, eye, and skin color?
    a. collagen
    b. elastin
    c. melanin
    d. keratin _____

62. What are melanocytes?
    a. dangerous bacteria that impede melanin production
    b. cells that produce skin pigment granules in the basal layer
    c. products that are unsafe to use because they deplete melanin
    d. cells that produce melanin within the horny and spiny layers _____

63. What are melanosomes?
    a. blood vessels dedicated to moving melanin through the body
    b. blotches on the skin where excess melanin is located
    c. pale patches on the skin where insufficient melanin is located
    d. pigment-carrying granules that produce melanin _____

64. What is true of the papillary layer of the skin?
    a. it is the top layer of the dermis
    b. it is the middle layer of the dermis
    c. it is the deepest layer of the dermis
    d. it is part of the epidermis _____

65. What is true of the reticular layer of the skin?
    a. it is part of the epidermis
    b. it is the deepest layer of the dermis
    c. it is the middle layer of the dermis
    d. it is the top layer of the dermis _____

CHAPTER 11—DISORDERS AND DISEASES OF THE SKIN

1. What term is used to describe any mark, wound, or abnormality?
   a. lesion
   b. papule
   c. cyst
   d. skin tag

   _____

2. What is leukoderma?
   a. flat, hairy spots on the skin
   b. light patches caused by destroyed pigment-producing cells
   c. brown or wine-colored discoloration
   d. thick scar resulting from excessive fibrous tissue

   _____

3. What is the term for a flat spot or discoloration of the skin, such as a freckle?
   a. pustule
   b. cyst
   c. macule
   d. stain

   _____

4. What is true of malignant melanoma?
   a. it is a benign form of skin cancer
   b. it is the least serious form of skin cancer
   c. it is a moderately serious form of skin cancer
   d. it is the most serious form of skin cancer

   _____

5. What condition is also known as melasma?
   a. hyperpigmentation
   b. hypopigmentation
   c. benign melanoma
   d. malignant melanoma

   _____

6. What is an example of epidermal cysts?
   a. scars
   b. milia
   c. boils
   d. blisters

   _____

7. What is another name for the acute inflammatory disorder miliaria rubra?
   a. prickly heat
   b. scabies
   c. rabies
   d. shingles

   _____

8. What term refers to a pigmented nevus?
   a. nodule
   b. vesicle
   c. papule
   d. mole

   _____

9. What are nodules?
   a. brown or wine-colored discolorations
   b. small bumps caused by conditions such as scar tissue or infections
   c. large blisters containing watery fluid
   d. clusters of boils

   _____

10. What is another name for a nevus?
    a. carbuncle
    c. birthmark
    b. wheal
    d. skin tag _____

11. What is a tubercle?
    a. open lesion on the skin or mucous membrane of the body
    b. abnormal rounded, solid lump larger than a papule
    c. yeast infection of the skin that inhibits melanin production
    d. another name for the contagious infection called ringworm _____

12. What is tinea versicolor?
    a. pigmentation disease characterized by white patches
    b. yeast infection of the skin that inhibits melanin production
    c. generic term for any kind of fungal infection
    d. severe oiliness of the skin _____

13. What is the common name for the contagious infection tinea corporis?
    a. ringworm
    c. rabies
    b. shingles
    d. scabies _____

14. What is the generic term for a fungal infection?
    a. miliaria
    c. verruca
    b. tinea
    d. barbae _____

15. What is the scientific term for couperose skin?
    a. tinea barbae
    c. telangiectasia
    b. tinea pedis
    d. pseudofolliculitis _____

16. What causes the skin to tan upon exposure to ultraviolet (UV) radiation?
    a. increase in pigmentation
    b. increase in blood circulation
    c. increase in lymph production
    d. increase in body temperature _____

17. What is a steatoma?
    a. brown or wine-colored discoloration
    b. sebaceous cyst of subcutaneous tumor filled with sebum
    c. brownish spot ranging in color from tan to bluish-black
    d. small, benign outgrowth of the skin that looks like a flap _____

18. What is the term for a brown or wine-colored discoloration?
    a. wen
    c. tan
    b. wheal
    d. stain _____

19. What is a characteristic of the form of skin cancer called squamous cell carcinoma?
    a. pearly translucency to fleshy color
    b. scaly red or pink papules or nodules
    c. dark purple splotches at the joints
    d. asymmetrical area and color variation   _____

20. What are skin tags?
    a. small, benign outgrowths of the skin that look like flaps
    b. dangerous manifestations of malignant melanoma
    c. thick scars resulting from excessive fibrous tissue
    d. decaying discharges from infected comedones   _____

21. What is rosacea?
    a. any skin with a naturally rose-hued color
    b. condition characterized by redness and dilation of blood vessels
    c. light-colored, raised mark on the skin formed after injury
    d. skin cream used for treating fair-skinned clients   _____

22. What is the term for flaky skin cells or any thin plate of epidermal flakes, dry or oily?
    a. vesicles   c. skin tags
    b. scales   d. papules   _____

23. What is a light-colored, slightly raised mark on the skin that is formed after an injury or lesion of the skin has healed?
    a. stain   c. tan
    b. scar   d. wheal   _____

24. What are sebaceous filaments?
    a. mainly solidified impactions of oil without the cell matter
    b. light-colored, slightly raised marks on the skin formed after injuries
    c. thin plates of epidermal flakes, such as excessive dandruff
    d. small clusters of papules caused by products used on the face   _____

25. What is an example of sebaceous hyperplasia?
    a. benign lesions frequently seen in oilier areas of the face
    b. solidified impactions of oil without the cell matter
    c. light-colored, slightly raised marks on the skin formed after injuries
    d. patches covered with white-silver scales   _____

26. What is acne?
    a. medical condition defined by an absence of melanin pigment
    b. chronic inflammatory skin disorder of the sebaceous glands
    c. excess inflammation from allergies and irritants
    d. foul-smelling perspiration, usually in the armpits or feet _____

27. What is acne excorciee?
    a. severe form of acne that is considered precancerous
    b. skin type of anyone who regularly gets acne lesions
    c. product that makes acne lesions vanish instantaneously
    d. disorder where clients purposely scrape off acne lesions _____

28. What are actinic keratoses?
    a. large blisters containing watery fluid that are similar to vesicles
    b. clusters of boils
    c. pink or flesh-colored precancerous lesions that result from sun damage
    d. closed, abnormally developed sacs _____

29. What is albinism?
    a. deficiency in perspiration
    b. dry, scaly skin resulting from sebum deficiency
    c. foul-smelling perspiration
    d. medical condition defined by an absence of melanin pigment _____

30. What is anhidrosis?
    a. deficiency in perspiration
    b. excessive perspiration
    c. foul-smelling perspiration
    d. bloody perspiration _____

31. What is asteatosis?
    a. medical condition defined by an absence of melanin pigment
    b. dry, scaly skin from sebum deficiency
    c. excess inflammation from allergies and irritants
    d. disorder where clients purposely scrape off acne lesions _____

32. What is the term for excess inflammation (dry skin, redness, itching) from allergies and irritants?
    a. squamous cell melanoma   c. atopic dermatitis
    b. contact dermatitis   d. basal cell melanoma _____

33. What is true of basal cell carcinoma?
    a. it is the least common type of skin cancer
    b. it is the least severe type of skin cancer
    c. it is the most serious type of skin cancer
    d. it is a benign form of skin cancer _____

70

34. What is the term for foul-smelling perspiration, usually in the armpits or on the feet?
    a. tinea pedis
    b. bromhidrosis
    c. asteatosis
    d. tinea barbae   ____

35. What is a bulla?
    a. mass of hardened sebum and skin cells in a hair follicle
    b. closed comedone
    c. open comedone
    d. large blister containing watery fluid that is larger than a vesicle   ____

36. What is hyperkeratosis?
    a. overproduction of pigment
    b. underproduction of pigment
    c. thickening of the skin caused by a mass of keratinized cells
    d. thinning of the skin caused by a lack of keratinized cells   ____

37. What is the term for the overproduction of pigment?
    a. hyperpigmentation
    b. superpigmentation
    c. metapigmentation
    d. hypopigmentation   ____

38. What is hypertrophy?
    a. abnormal growth
    b. normal growth
    c. abnormal perspiration
    d. normal perspiration   ____

39. What is hypopigmentation?
    a. excess of pigment
    b. injection of pigment
    c. surgical removal of pigment
    d. lack of pigment   ____

40. What is impetigo?
    a. light, abnormal patches that are the result of congenital defects
    b. scar tissue resulting from excessive growth of fibrous tissue
    c. contagious bacterial infection marked by clusters of small blisters
    d. redness and bumpiness in the cheeks caused by blocked follicles   ____

41. What is a thick scar resulting from excessive growth of fibrous tissue (collagen)?
    a. stain
    b. keloid
    c. wheal
    d. wen   ____

42. What is a keratoma?
    a. thick scar resulting from excessive growth of fibrous tissue
    b. open comedone
    c. closed comedone
    d. acquired, thickened patch of epidermis   ____

43. What are abnormally thick build-ups of cells?
    a. keratoses   c. vesicles
    b. keloids   d. papules   ____

44. What is keratosis pilaris?
    a. acquired, thickened patch of epidermis
    b. redness and bumpiness in the cheeks caused by blocked
       follicles
    c. most malignant form of skin cancer
    d. least malignant form of skin cancer   ____

45. What is the scientific name for a freckle?
    a. vitiligo   c. melasma
    b. macule   d. lentigo   ____

46. What are secondary lesions?
    a. benign outgrowths of the skin that look like flaps
    b. skin damage that changes the structure of tissues or organs
    c. thick scars resulting from excessive growth of fibrous tissue
    d. brown or wine-colored discolorations   ____

47. What is seborrheic dermatitis?
    a. rare form of rosacea   c. rare form of eczema
    b. common form of rosacea   d. common form of eczema   ____

48. What is severe oiliness of the skin called?
    a. dermatitis   c. eczema
    b. seborrhea   d. rosacea   ____

49. Where in the face does the acne-like condition perioral dermatitis
    manifest?
    a. forehead   c. nose
    b. chin   d. mouth   ____

50. What is a characteristic of primary lesions?
    a. brownish spots ranging in color from tan to bluish-black
    b. subcutaneous tumors filled with sebum
    c. infection with ringed, red pattern with elevated ridges
    d. flat, nonpalpable changes in skin color such as maculae
       or patches   ____

51. What is the term for persistent itching?
    a. dermatitis   c. hepatitis
    b. pruitis   d. mitosis   _____

52. What is the common name for pseudofolliculitis?
    a. skin tags   c. freckles
    b. razor bumps   d. pimples   _____

53. What is a characteristic of psoriasis?
    a. red patches covered with white-silver scales
    b. subcutaneous tumors filled with sebum
    c. flat, nonpalpable changes in skin color such as maculae or
       patches
    d. benign outgrowths of the skin that look like flaps   _____

54. What is a pustule?
    a. inflamed wheal   c. irritated vesicle
    b. irritated wen   d. inflamed papule   _____

55. When someone has retention hyperkeratinosis, what builds up
    and fails to shed from the follicles as happens in normal skin?
    a. sebum   c. perspiration
    b. dead skin cells   d. hairs   _____

56. What is the term for a cluster of boils?
    a. wheal   c. comedone
    b. wen   d. carbuncle   _____

57. What is the common name for chloasma?
    a. razor bumps   c. liver spots
    b. skin tags   d. fine wrinkles   _____

58. What is true of a comedogenic product?
    a. it has no adverse effects on the skin whatsoever
    b. it tends to clog follicles and cause a buildup of
       dead skin cells
    c. it helps clear up comedones quickly and safely
    d. this sort of product should not be used on human skin   _____

59. What is a comedone?
    a. cluster of boils
    b. large blister containing watery fluid
    c. mass of hardened sebum and skin cells in a hair follicle
    d. pink or flesh-colored precancerous lesion   _____

60. What is the common name for the very contagious infection conjunctivitis?
    a. ringworm
    b. pinkeye
    c. rabies
    d. scabies
    ____

61. What is contact dermatitis?
    a. foul-smelling perspiration
    b. the effect when two skin disorders connect with each other
    c. an inflammation caused by contact with a substance or chemical
    d. excessive perspiration
    ____

62. What is crust an accumulation of?
    a. sweat and dirt
    b. water and salt
    c. blood and lymph
    d. sebum and pus
    ____

63. What is a closed, abnormally developed sac containing fluid, infection, or other matter above and below the skin?
    a. vesicle
    b. cyst
    c. comedone
    d. papule
    ____

64. What is dermatitis?
    a. excessive oiliness of the skin
    b. excessive dryness of the skin
    c. any cancerous condition of the skin
    d. any inflammatory condition of the skin
    ____

65. What type of physician specializes in treating skin disorders and diseases?
    a. dermatologist
    b. physiologist
    c. esthetician
    d. cosmetologist
    ____

66. What is a papule?
    a. another name for the skin malformations called birthmarks
    b. tumors caused by conditions such as scar tissue and infections
    c. small elevation of the skin that contains fluid and may develop pus
    d. itchy, swollen lesion caused by a blow, insect bite, or sting
    ____

67. What are **NOT** examples of wheals?
    a. hives
    b. mosquito bites
    c. uticaria
    d. pustules
    ____

68. What is vitiligo?
    a. contagious skin condition
    b. allergic reaction to strong chemicals in cleaning products
    c. total absence of pigmentation
    d. pigmentation disease characterized by white patches
    ____

69. What is a small blister or sac containing clear fluid?
   a. vesicle
   c. melanoma
   b. carbuncle
   d. wen
   _____

70. What is the common name for the hypertrophy of the papillae and epidermis known as a verruca?
   a. wheal
   c. wen
   b. wart
   d. wick
   _____

71. What is another term for varicose veins?
   a. primary lesions
   c. secondary lesions
   b. vascular lesions
   d. foreign lesions
   _____

72. What is the term for vascular dilation of blood vessels?
   a. cardiodilation
   c. plasmadilation
   b. pulmodilation
   d. vasodilation
   _____

73. What is the common name for urticaria, which is caused by an allergic reaction form the body's histamine production?
   a. pinkeye
   c. scabies
   b. ringworm
   d. hives
   _____

74. What accompanies an ulcer in addition to a loss of skin depth?
   a. pus
   c. lymph
   b. blood
   d. sebum
   _____

75. What is the term for an abnormal cell mass that results from excessive cell multiplication and varies in size, shape, and color?
   a. tumor
   c. skin tag
   b. comedone
   d. razor bump
   _____

76. What is eczema?
   a. pigmentation disease characterized by white patches
   b. inflammatory, painful itching disease of the skin
   c. yeast infection on the skin that inhibits melanin production
   d. contagious infection that forms a ringed, red pattern
   _____

77. What is edema?
   a. any inflammatory condition of the skin
   b. swelling caused by a fluid imbalance in cells
   c. brownish spot ranging in color from tan to bluish-black
   d. closed, abnormally developed sac containing fluid or other matter
   _____

78. What is erythema?
    a. oiliness caused by inflammation
    b. redness caused by inflammation
    c. dryness caused by inflammation
    d. pain caused by inflammation ____

79. What is excoriation?
    a. lesion caused by an allergic reaction
    b. skin sore or abrasion produced by scratching or scraping
    c. type of contagious fungal infection
    d. common side effect of blood-thinning medications ____

80. What is a fissure?
    a. crack in the skin that penetrates the dermis
    b. opening, such as a pore, through which fluids escape
       the body
    c. another name for a follicle
    d. another name for an orifice ____

81. What is folliculitis?
    a. excessive hair growth
    b. insufficient hair growth
    c. inflammation of the hair follicles
    d. another term for razor bumps ____

82. What is true of herpes simplex 1?
    a. it causes fever blisters and cold sores
    b. it causes hepatitis
    c. it is the virus that causes AIDS
    d. it is always a terminal condition ____

83. What is the common name for the painful viral infection herpes
    zoster?
    a. scabies   c. pinkeye
    b. shingles   d. ringworm ____

84. What is hyperhidrosis?
    a. insufficient perspiration
    b. excessive perspiration
    c. foul-smelling perspiration
    d. sweet-smelling perspiration ____

85. What part of the body is affected by herpes simplex 2?
    a. face   c. feet
    b. hair   d. genitals ____

CHAPTER 12—SKIN ANALYSIS

1. What is a characteristic of seborrhea?
   a. oily skin
   b. dry skin
   c. flaky skin
   d. scaly skin   ____

2. What are intrinsic factors?
   a. nutritional qualities in the food that we eat
   b. factors related to our body's internal health
   c. factors related to the body's external health
   d. unavoidable environmental factors in a geographic area   ____

3. What are extrinsic factors?
   a. health factors inside the body
   b. health factors outside the body
   c. circulatory health factors
   d. genetic health factors   ____

4. What is true of sun damage?
   a. it is a myth that sun exposure damages the skin
   b. sun damage is only a minor factor in the overall health of the skin
   c. it is the main intrinsic cause of aging
   d. it is the main extrinsic cause of aging   ____

5. What does dehydrated skin lack?
   a. oil
   b. water
   c. lymph
   d. sebum   ____

6. What is **NOT** an indicator of dry skin?
   a. flaky appearance
   b. tight feeling
   c. absorbs product quickly
   d. absorbs product slowly   ____

7. What is true of normal skin?
   a. it has a good oil-water balance
   b. it has a poor oil-water balance
   c. it has no oil content
   d. it has no water content   ____

8. Where on the face of a client with normal skin are follicles smaller to medium?
   a. on the forehead
   b. on the chin
   c. on the edge of the T-zone by the nose
   d. beneath the eyes   ____

9. What skin type is associated with the treatment goals of maintenance and preventative care?
   a. combination
   b. dry
   c. normal
   d. oily
   ____

10. What skin type is associated with the treatment goals of using occlusive products to reduce transepidermal water loss (TWL)?
   a. combination
   b. dry
   c. normal
   d. oily
   ____

11. What skin type is associated with the treatment goals of extra cleansing and exfoliating?
   a. combination
   b. dry
   c. oily
   d. normal
   ____

12. What skin type is associated with the treatment goals of soothing, drying, and protecting?
   a. dry
   b. normal
   c. oily
   d. sensitive
   ____

13. Where on the face of a client with combination skin are the follicles medium to larger?
   a. on the forehead
   b. outside the T-zone on the cheeks
   c. outside the mouth on the chin
   d. on the nose
   ____

14. What causes actinic aging?
   a. sun exposure
   b. excessive moisture
   c. improper shaving
   d. inappropriate use of drying products
   ____

15. What does alipidic skin lack?
   a. water
   b. oil
   c. lymph
   d. oxygen
   ____

16. What are contraindications?
   a. instructions for the use of products
   b. instructions for the use of tools
   c. factors that prohibit a treatment
   d. factors that indicate a treatment will be beneficial
   ____

17. What type of skin is indicated by redness and is the result of distended capillaries from weakening of the capillary walls?
    a. dry
    b. combination
    c. oily
    d. couperose
    ____

18. What does the Fitzpatrick Scale measure?
    a. skin's ability to tolerate sun exposure
    b. skin's ability to tolerate water exposure
    c. skin's ability to absorb products applied to the epidermis
    d. skin's ability to recover from injection punctures
    ____

19. What does the term "keratosis" refer to?
    a. abnormally thick buildup of cells
    b. area with insufficient cells
    c. bruise caused by injury
    d. acne caused by poor skin care
    ____

20. What do occlusive products reduce?
    a. water loss
    b. heat loss
    c. pigmentation loss
    d. skin density loss
    ____

21. When should you analyze the client's skin type and conditions?
    a. before performing services
    b. while performing services
    c. after performing services
    d. while scheduling the client's next appointment
    ____

22. What type on the Fitzpatrick Scale is a person with Middle Eastern skin, dark or black hair, and brown eyes?
    a. type II
    b. type III
    c. type IV
    d. type V
    ____

23. What are the general characteristics of type III skin on the Fitzpatrick Scale?
    a. fair-skinned; light eyes; light hair
    b. very fair; blond or red hair; light colored eyes; freckles common
    c. fair skin; varied eye color; varied hair color
    d. Mediterranean Caucasian skin; dark brown hair
    ____

24. What is type VI skin on the Fitzpatrick Scale?
    a. pale skin
    b. fair skin
    c. Mediterranean skin
    d. black skin
    ____

25. What is true of type I skin on the Fitzpatrick Scale?
    a. always burns
    b. often burns
    c. sometimes burns
    d. never burns

26. What is true of type VI skin on the Fitzpatrick Scale?
    a. always burns
    b. often burns
    c. sometimes burns
    d. may never burn

27. What evaluates photodamage based on wrinkling categorized by age?
    a. Fitzpatrick Scale
    b. McCormick Scale
    c. Glogau Scale
    d. Richter Scale

28. What makes one person's skin darker than another person's skin?
    a. greater amounts of melanin
    b. lesser amounts of melanin
    c. greater amounts of lymph
    d. lesser amounts of lymph

29. What skin type is more likely to have a greater problem with hyperpigmentation than the other skin types?
    a. pale
    b. fair
    c. medium
    d. dark

30. What is a characteristic of actinic keratosis?
    a. oily patch that does not abate after thorough cleansing
    b. rough area resulting from sun exposure, sometimes peeling off
    c. cluster of comedones surrounded by a field of redness
    d. irritated area exuding pus through cracks in the skin

31. What is a characteristic of erythmea?
    a. irregular heartbeat
    b. irregular respiration
    c. redness caused by inflammation
    d. pain caused by swelling

32. What term indicates that a treatment is prohibited for a particular client?
    a. contravened
    b. contradicted
    c. contraindicated
    d. contrasted

33. What are skin types?
    a. medical terms differentiating between ethnicities
    b. esthetician terms used to identify common skin conditions
    c. classifications that describe a person's genetic skin type
    d. pharmaceutical terms referring to thickness of the skin

34. What determines a person's skin type?
    a. genetics and ethnicity   c. diet and exercise
    b. personality and temperament   d. personal stress level   _____

35. What can be indicated by the size of the pores in the T-zone and
    throughout the face?
    a. skin type   c. internal body temperature
    b. blood pressure   d. overall health   _____

36. What is **NOT** one of the four skin types?
    a. combination   c. sensitive
    b. dry   d. oily   _____

37. What skin types require proper cleansing, exfoliating, and
    hydrating?
    a. normal and oily   c. normal and combination
    b. dry and oily   d. all skin types   _____

38. What is a characteristic of dry skin?
    a. large follicles   c. normal follicles
    b. small follicles   d. closed follicles   _____

39. What type of skin needs extra care because it does not produce
    enough oil?
    a. dry   c. normal
    b. oily   d. sensitive   _____

40. What is a characteristic of dry skin?
    a. tight feeling, slightly rough   c. large, spread-out follicles
    b. loose feeling, soft to the touch d. large, sebum-filled follicles   _____

41. What is another name for oily skin?
    a. wet skin   c. lymphatic skin
    b. moist skin   d. lipidic skin   _____

42. What is a characteristic of oily skin?
    a. extremely small follicles throughout the face
    b. follicles that are visible or larger over most of the face
    c. follicles that are large only on the chin
    d. follicles that are large only on the cheeks   _____

43. What is oily skin prone to because pores get clogged with oil?
    a. hyperpigmentation   c. blemishes
    b. hypopigmentation   d. vellus hair   _____

44. What should you try to balance in all skin types?
   a. skin color
   b. barrier function
   c. skin thickness
   d. circulation
   ____

45. What type of skin ages more slowly than the other types?
   a. dry skin
   b. oily skin
   c. normal
   d. sensitive
   ____

46. What is a characteristic of sensitive skin?
   a. easy absorption of product
   b. small follicles
   c. fragile, thin skin and redness
   d. large follicles
   ____

47. What type of skin can be difficult to treat because of its low tolerance for products and stimulation?
   a. oily
   b. combination
   c. normal
   d. sensitive
   ____

48. What type on the Fitzpatrick Scale is a person with very fair skin, blond or red hair, light colored eyes, and possibly freckles?
   a. type I
   b. type II
   c. type III
   d. type IV
   ____

49. What type on the Fitzpatrick Scale is a person with Mediterranean Caucasian skin and dark brown hair?
   a. type II
   b. type III
   c. type IV
   d. type V
   ____

50. What type on the Fitzpatrick Scale is a person with fair skin, light eyes, and light hair?
   a. type I
   b. type II
   c. type III
   d. type IV
   ____

CHAPTER 13—SKIN CARE PRODUCTS: CHEMISTRY, INGREDIENTS, AND SELECTION

1. What are botanicals made from?
   a. plants and herbs
   b. chemicals
   c. animal fats
   d. recycled plastic

   _____

2. What is **NOT** among the components of lipids?
   a. phospholipids
   b. ceramides
   c. botanicals
   d. sterols

   _____

3. What is **NOT** something from which healing agents are made?
   a. recycled plastics
   b. licorice
   c. aloe
   d. chamomile

   _____

4. What is a possible advantage of synthetic ingredients over natural ingredients?
   a. fewer allergic reactions
   b. shorter shelf life
   c. less environmental impact
   d. decreased chemical content

   _____

5. When is a manufacturer responsible for a client's allergic reaction to a product?
   a. when the product is purchased in bulk and repackaged by the salon
   b. when the product is used as an ingredient in a salon mixture
   c. when the product is taken directly from the manufacturer's packaging
   d. when the client ignores warnings on the product's label

   _____

6. When is the salon responsible for a client's allergic reaction to a product?
   a. when the client buys the product directly form the manufacturer
   b. when the product is purchased in bulk and repackaged by the salon
   c. when the client ignores warnings on the product's label
   d. when the product is taken directly from the manufacturer's packaging

   _____

7. What is true of organic labeling standards for cosmetics in the United States?
   a. these labeling standards are numerous and strict
   b. these labeling standards are few and lenient
   c. there are no such standards in the United States
   d. standards from other countries are enforced in the United States ____

8. What is **NOT** an area requiring approval from the Food and Drug Administration (FDA)?
   a. cosmetics manufacturing   c. cosmetics labeling
   b. cosmetics safety   d. cosmetics claims ____

9. What term refers to skin-freshening lotions with a low alcohol content?
   a. moisturizers   c. fresheners
   b. antibiotics   d. conditioners ____

10. What is **NOT** among the purposes of functional ingredients in cosmetic products?
   a. allowing products to spread
   b. giving products body and texture
   c. making products affordable
   d. giving products specific form ____

11. What is **NOT** true of glycerin?
   a. it is formed by a decomposition of oils or fats
   b. it is a very weak water binder
   c. it is an excellent skin softener
   d. it is an excellent humectant ____

12. What term refers to an exfoliating cream that is rubbed off the skin?
   a. humectant   c. gommage
   b. emulsifier   d. paraben ____

13. What is grapeseed extract?
   a. powerful antioxidant with soothing properties
   b. powerful antioxidant with stimulating properties
   c. powerful exfoliant with soothing properties
   d. powerful exfoliant with stimulating properties ____

14. What are hydrators?
   a. machines used to apply water to the skin's surface
   b. machines used to extract water from the skin's surface
   c. ingredients that attract water to the skin's surface
   d. ingredients that repel water from the skin's surface ____

15. What are alpha hydroxy acids?
   a. products that exfoliate by loosening bonds between dead cells
   b. products that exfoliate by tightening bonds between living cells
   c. the active ingredients in most acne-treatment medications
   d. the active ingredients in most dandruff-control shampoos ____

16. What type of product does **NOT** sometimes include alcohol?
   a. perfume
   b. lotion
   c. astringent
   d. paraffin mask ____

17. What is **NOT** true of aloe vera?
   a. it is the most popular botanical used in cosmetic formulations
   b. it is the least popular botanical used in cosmetic formulations
   c. it is an emollient and film-forming gum resin
   d. it has hydrating and softening qualities, among others ____

18. Where in the body is alpha liponic acid found?
   a. every cell
   b. nerve cells
   c. blood cells
   d. striated muscle cells ____

19. What is an ampoule?
   a. small, sealed vial
   b. needle used for injections
   c. popular botanical cream
   d. family of chemical products ____

20. What is aromatherapy?
   a. practice of focusing massage on the nose and nostrils
   b. therapeutic use of plant aromas and essential oils
   c. therapeutic use of scented candles in the treatment room
   d. practice of focusing acupuncture on the nose and nostrils ____

21. What are astringents?
   a. cotton pads used to dab excess sebum from the surface of the skin
   b. cotton pads used to dab excess lymph from the surface of the skin
   c. oil-laden liquids used to increase the oiliness of the skin
   d. liquids that help remove excess oil on the skin ____

22. What is **NOT** true of benzoyl peroxide?
   a. it is commonly used for blemishes
   b. it is commonly used for acne
   c. it is a drying agent
   d. it is a type of alpha hydroxy acid ____

23. What is glycerin?
    a. astringent   c. exfoliant
    b. binder   d. antibiotic   _____

24. What are ingredients derived from plants called?
    a. chemicals   c. pentacostals
    b. pharmaceuticals   d. botanicals   _____

25. What are ceramides?
    a. astringents that have moisturizing and antibacterial
       properties
    b. family of lipid materials that are part of the intercellular
       matrix
    c. bacteria that cause itching in the surface of the skin
    d. clusters of dead skin cells that clog follicles and cause
       comedones   _____

26. What plant extract has calming and soothing properties?
    a. blackcurrant   c. ginseng
    b. chamomile   d. honeybush   _____

27. What is jojoba?
    a. oil extracted from the acorns that grow on oak trees
    b. oil extracted from the bean-like seeds of a desert shrub
    c. exfoliating agent made from the gritty sand of tropical
       beaches
    d. moisturizing agent made from Pacific Ocean seaweed   _____

28. What is another term for exfoliation?
    a. sloughing   c. excoriation
    b. binding   d. emulsification   _____

29. What are lakes?
    a. insoluble pigments   c. botanical emulsifiers
    b. botanical moisturizers   d. insoluble antioxidants   _____

30. What is an emollient with moisturizing properties and also an
    emulsifier with high water absorption capabilities?
    a. chamomile   c. papaya
    b. jojoba   d. lanolin   _____

31. What products coat the skin and reduce friction?
    a. lubricants   c. emulsifiers
    b. antioxidants   d. acids   _____

32. What is **NOT** true of polymers?
    a. they are chemical compounds
    b. they are botanicals
    c. they are formed by small molecules
    d. they release substances at a microscopically controlled rate ____

33. What is potassium hydroxide?
    a. strong alkali used in soaps and creams
    b. weak alkali used in soaps and creams
    c. strong acid used in soaps and creams
    d. weak acid used in soaps and creams ____

34. What function do preservatives perform?
    a. give products the desired color, shape, and form
    b. give products the desired efficacy and strength
    c. activate products once they are applied to the skin
    d. inhibit the growth of microorganisms ____

35. What is the vitamin of which retinol is the natural form?
    a. vitamin A   c. vitamin C
    b. vitamin B   d. vitamin D ____

36. What is **NOT** a natural source of salicylic acid?
    a. jojoba   c. willow bark
    b. sweet birch   d. wintergreen ____

37. What does the term "comedogenicity" refer to?
    a. tendency of some ethnicities to have more comedones
       than others
    b. scientific study of the genetics of comedones
    c. tendency of any substance to trigger the rise of blackheads
    d. tendency of any substance to inhibit the rise of blackheads ____

38. What is **NOT** true of tissue respiratory factor (TRF)?
    a. it is an anti-inflammatory ingredient
    b. it is a natural antibiotic
    c. it is a moisturizing ingredient
    d. it is derived from yeast cells ____

39. What vitamin has **NOT** been used in skin care products as an antioxidant?
    a. vitamin A   c. vitamin C
    b. vitamin B   d. vitamin E ____

40. What are liposomes?
    a. open-lipid bilayer spheres
    b. open-lipid unilayer spores
    c. closed-lipid bilayer spheres
    d. closed-lipid unilayer spores _____

41. What is mechanical exfoliation?
    a. physical method of rubbing dead cells off the skin
    b. use of machines to push product deeper into the skin
    c. physical method of drawing pus from a whitehead
    d. use of machines to draw pus from a whitehead _____

42. What is mineral oil?
    a. lubricant derived from petroleum
    b. antioxidant derived from petroleum
    c. lubricant derived from sebum
    d. antioxidant derived from sebum _____

43. What are mucopolysaccharides?
    a. irritated mucous membranes
    b. healthy mucous membranes
    c. carbohydrate-lipid complexes
    d. carbohydrate-lymph complexes _____

44. What is the strongest of our five senses?
    a. taste   c. smell
    b. touch   d. sight _____

45. What is papaya used for?
    a. exfoliation   c. hydration
    b. moisturizing   d. pigmentation _____

46. What is **NOT** an industry that commonly uses parabens?
    a. cosmetic   c. food
    b. pharmaceutical   d. aeronautic _____

47. What are peptides?
    a. chains of red blood cells   c. chains of fibroblasts
    b. chains of white blood cells d. chains of amino acids _____

48. What are performance ingredients?
    a. ingredients included to elongate the shelf life of products
    b. ingredients used to give products distinct shape and texture
    c. ingredients that cause actual changes in the appearance of
       the skin
    d. ingredients that stimulate blood circulation and increase energy _____

49. What is **NOT** true of petroleum jelly?
    a. it is commonly used after laser surgery
    b. it holds water in the skin
    c. it is an occlusive agent
    d. it dehydrates the skin ____

50. What term refers to the use of plant extracts for therapeutic benefits?
    a. arboratherapy   c. ecotherapy
    b. green therapy   d. phyotherapy ____

51. What is a chelating agent?
    a. chemical added to improve the thickness of a product
    b. chemical added to improve the efficacy of the preservative
    c. chemical added to soften the aroma of a product
    d. chemical added to increase the grit of a product ____

52. What do clay masks do as they dry and tighten?
    a. seal follicles
    b. rupture comedones
    c. extract facial hairs
    d. draw impurities to the surface ____

53. What is coenzyme Q10?
    a. antioxidant   c. preservative
    b. exfoliant   d. emulsifier ____

54. What is the term for substances such as mineral dyes that give products color?
    a. color additives   c. colorants
    b. color ingredients   d. chromophores ____

55. What term refers to products intended to improve the skin's health and appearance?
    a. cosmetics   c. epidermals
    b. cosmeceuticals   d. estheticals ____

56. What are detergents a type of?
    a. surfactant   c. antioxidant
    b. emollient   d. exfoliant ____

57. What do emulsifiers cause to mix in order to form an emulsion?
    a. oil and lymph   c. lymph and water
    b. oil and water   d. lymph and sebum ____

58. What is exfoliation?
    a. careful removal of a clay or paraffin mask from the skin
    b. thorough cleansing of the skin with soap and hot water
    c. peeling or sloughing of the outer layer of the skin
    d. use of chemicals to reduce the size of the inner layers of the skin _____

59. What are fatty acids?
    a. excessive sebum discharges common in overweight clients
    b. excessive lymph discharges common in overweight clients
    c. antioxidant ingredients derived solely from animal fats
    d. lubricant ingredients derived from plant oils or animal fats _____

60. What function do fragrances perform?
    a. giving products their color
    b. giving products their scent
    c. giving products their taste
    d. giving products their texture _____

Part 4: Esthetics

CHAPTER 14—THE TREATMENT ROOM

1. What should you wash your hands with before touching clean
   supplies?
   a. soap and warm water
   b. chemical disinfectant
   c. autoclave steam
   d. harsh exfoliant   ____

2. What should you do with single-use items as you prepare for a
   treatment?
   a. place them on a countertop in descending size order
   b. set them on a clean towel in the order they will be used
   c. place them on a countertop in ascending size order
   d. set them on a clean towel in order of importance   ____

3. When should you clean and disinfect the nail brush you keep in
   your room to scrub your nails and hands?
   a. after each use
   b. twice each day
   c. whenever you take a break
   d. only at the end of each day   ____

4. What should you do to accommodate the fact that some clients
   have never received facial or waxing treatments before?
   a. remain silent while clients figure out for themselves how to
      do things
   b. ask the receptionist to educate clients before treatments
   c. prepare a brochure explaining what you expect from each client
   d. explain to the client where to put belongings and how to
      put on the wrap   ____

5. Why should you wear gloves for all decontamination procedures?
   a. only to prevent contamination
   b. only to protect your skin from strong chemicals
   c. to prevent contamination and protect your skin from strong
      chemicals
   d. it is not necessary to wear gloves for all decontamination procedures ____

6. What is true of butterfly pads?
   a. they are superior to round pads in all respects
   b. they will not fall off the eyes as easily as round pads
   c. butterfly pads are only useful for clients with sensitive skin
   d. butterfly pads are only useful for clients with couperose skin ____

7. When in the procedure for making cleansing pads do you squeeze out excess water?
   a. at the beginning
   b. at the end
   c. in the middle
   d. anytime you wish ____

8. How many facial treatments can you perform with four to six cleansing pads?
   a. one
   b. three
   c. five
   d. seven ____

9. When should you consider using a roll of cotton to make cleansing pads?
   a. when you are too tired to make a trip to the supply room
   b. when your client has oily skin
   c. when prepackaged esthetic wipes or sponges are unavailable
   d. when your client has dry skin ____

10. What should happen before the client leaves your treatment area?
    a. payment
    b. rebooking
    c. retail purchases
    d. product recommendations ____

11. When in your end-of-day procedure should you put on a fresh pair of gloves?
    a. at the beginning
    b. at the end
    c. whenever you realize you're about to touch something dirty
    d. whenever you realize you're about to touch something wet ____

12. What can you do to prevent mildew from growing in the laundry hamper?
    a. leave the hamper open so fresh air circulates
    b. take wet laundry out of the hamper once each day
    c. disinfect the hamper after removing all dirty laundry
    d. spray the hamper with disinfectant whenever it gets full ____

13. What should you do once you've escorted the client to the reception desk?
    a. hold out your hand for a tip
    b. write up a service ticket
    c. watch the client make payment
    d. ensure the client buys retail products ____

14. What do paper towels, tissues for blotting the face, and vinyl gloves have in common?
    a. they are multi-use items
    b. they are single-use items
    c. they are disinfecting products
    d. they are cleansing products ____

15. What piece of salon furniture is also known as an operator's stool?
    a. receptionist's chair
    b. esthetician's chair
    c. manager's chair
    d. client's chair _____

16. What is a sharps container?
    a. disinfectant-filled jar in which fresh hair shears are stored
    b. plastic case in which unused injectables are stored
    c. biohazard container for disposable needles and anything sharp
    d. special wastebasket for breakable items such as glass _____

17. What is a dispensary?
    a. drawer at the reception desk for storing retail products
    b. printing machine at your station that produces service tickets
    c. room or area used for mixing products and storing supplies
    d. another name for the pharmacy closest to your salon _____

18. What are implements?
    a. tools used by technicians
    b. ingrown hairs
    c. contraindications
    d. garments worn by clients _____

19. What does the "S" stand for in the acronym LOHAS?
    a. superiority
    b. seniority
    c. sustainability
    d. susceptibility _____

20. What does "sustainability" mean?
    a. acquiring enough goods to provide services for one year
    b. meeting the needs of the present without compromising the future
    c. building a client base that ensures an annual increase of profits
    d. compromising the future to ensure that present needs are met _____

21. What is facilitated by planning and preparing a well-stocked and organized treatment room?
    a. only functioning efficiently
    b. only providing good service
    c. perfect treatment results
    d. functioning efficiently and providing good service _____

22. Why is it important for estheticians/students to maintain clean treatment rooms?
    a. only client safety
    b. only compliance with laws
    c. client safety and compliance with laws
    d. cleaning treatment rooms is not the job of estheticians/students _____

23. What is a benefit of being prepared?
    a. you never encounter surprises
    b. you never have problems at work
    c. you project a calm, confident image
    d. you do everything well _____

24. When in the process of performing services do you plan and prepare the treatment room?
    a. at the beginning
    b. at the end
    c. once the client arrives
    d. once the treatment is underway _____

25. What are criteria for determining that a treatment table is large enough?
    a. large enough to accommodate clients, suitable for body waxing
    b. any size that fits into the treatment room is acceptable
    c. the only criteria is being large enough to accommodate clients
    d. the only criteria is being suitable for body waxing _____

26. What is the function of a magnifying lamp or light?
    a. directing LED beams
    b. analyzing the skin and performing detail work such as tweezing
    c. heating up product for deeper penetration into the dermis
    d. blocking LED beams _____

27. What can you do to accommodate walk-ins or unexpected requests?
    a. keep massage oil on your hands
    b. keep water running all day
    c. keep wax heaters on all day
    d. avoid taking breaks or lunches _____

28. What is **NOT** a salon area in which supplies are regularly kept?
    a. work station
    c. reception desk
    b. treatment room
    d. dispensary _____

29. What should you use to disperse products from jars?
    a. fingers
    c. tongs
    b. scissors
    d. spatulas _____

30. What should you have among your facial supplies in order to provide neck support for the client?
    a. wood block the size of a brick   c. medical neck brace
    b. pillow or rolled hand towel   d. thick turtleneck sweater   ____

31. What should you **NEVER** put beneath the bed linens?
    a. plastic sheeting   c. electric blankets
    b. paper for hygienic protection   d. clients   ____

32. How long, approximately, is required for pre-heating of towel warmers and steamers?
    a. five minutes   c. 30 minutes
    b. 15 minutes   d. 60 minutes   ____

33. When should you check the water level on the steamer?
    a. before preheating and regularly thereafter
    b. only before preheating
    c. only regularly throughout the day
    d. checking the water level is unnecessary   ____

34. What is true of distilled water?
    a. it should never be used in steamers
    b. it is the only type of water that should be used in steamers
    c. it is no better for steamers than any other type of water
    d. it should only be used in steamers if tap water is unavailable   ____

35. Why should you place a blanket over the clean linens that you place on the treatment table?
    a. only in order to keep the client warm
    b. in order to keep the client warm and comfortable
    c. only in order to keep the client comfortable
    d. in order to cut down how often linens must be cleaned   ____

CHAPTER 15—FACIAL TREATMENTS

1. What is a food or drink that does **NOT** aggravate rosacea?
   a. milk
   b. wine
   c. beer
   d. heavily spiced food
   ____

2. What skin condition can be prevented by staying out of the sun and wearing protective clothing and sunscreen daily?
   a. vitiligo
   b. hyperpigmentation
   c. hypopigmentation
   d. albinism
   ____

3. What does it mean if a client says that extractions are painful?
   a. client needs to get over his or her low pain threshold
   b. extractions should never be performed on this client
   c. you should immediately ask a manager to review your technique
   d. extraction method being used is probably too rough and forceful
   ____

4. What is **NOT** among the environmental aggravators that clients with acne should avoid?
   a. dirt
   b. grease
   c. humidity
   d. water
   ____

5. What procedure should you recommend that clients with acne add to their home care twice per week?
   a. enzyme peel
   b. clay mask
   c. therapeutic sun exposure
   d. aggressive massage
   ____

6. What are finger cots?
   a. trays filled with lotion for softening the skin of the fingertips
   b. wood slats strapped to the fingers to hold them rigid during treatment
   c. an industry term referring to each individual "sleeve" of a glove
   d. individual finger "gloves" used for extractions
   ____

7. What will you be able to perform easily and efficiently once you understand the angle of the various follicles in the different locations on the skin?
   a. enzyme peels
   b. extractions
   c. clay masks
   d. product application
   ____

8. When in the extraction process is a healing mask beneficial?
   a. before any extractions begin
   b. midway through the extractions
   c. after all extractions are done
   d. the day after extractions _____

9. What is **NOT** one of the beneficial effects that warmth has on skin?
   a. softens the follicles
   b. promotes effective cleansing
   c. decreases circulation
   d. prepares skin for extractions _____

10. What is **NOT** a risk associated with keeping hot towels on the skin for too long?
    a. overmoisturization
    b. overstimulation
    c. redness
    d. irritation _____

11. What is extraction?
    a. plucking hairs with tweezers
    b. manually removing impurities and comedones from follicles
    c. reducing excess hair from nostrils with a nose trimmer
    d. chemically extracting pigment _____

12. What is **NOT** one of the functions of a treatment mask?
    a. hydrating the skin
    b. rejuvenating the skin
    c. drawing out impurities
    d. loosening the skin _____

13. When in the facial process should a calming, hydrating mask be applied?
    a. anytime
    b. only at the beginning
    c. only at the end
    d. never _____

14. What becomes trapped under a paraffin mask and promotes penetration of ingredients deeper into the skin?
    a. heat
    b. moisture
    c. hydrogen
    d. nitrogen _____

15. Why should you offer clients water after performing services?
    a. to advertise the brand of water
    b. to add an item to the client's bill
    c. to increase your tip
    d. to facilitate rehydration _____

16. What should you do at the end of the service?
    a. perform a skin analysis
    b. book the client's next appointment
    c. perform the client consultation
    d. show the client around the salon _____

17. Why should you apply product moderately?
    a. any excess product you use is deducted from your paycheck
    b. you don't want to be the reason the salon runs out of a product
    c. most products are superconcentrated
    d. too much of a good thing can counteract benefits _____

18. What should you do if you are having a bad day?
    a. call in sick to work   c. avoid needy clients
    b. keep it to yourself   d. vent to your coworkers _____

19. What is **NOT** among the reasons clients should arrive 15 minutes prior to appointments?
    a. fill out the consultation form
    b. get into a robe
    c. help you prep the treatment room
    d. prepare for their treatment _____

20. When should the client be shown the area where he or she can change clothes and store any belongings?
    a. only when the client asks to see the area
    b. only if the treatment room is too small for these purposes
    c. at the end of the appointment
    d. immediately upon arrival in the salon _____

21. What should female clients be instructed to remove before a facial treatment?
    a. panties   c. garter belt
    b. bra   d. stockings _____

22. What sort of fabric is **MOST** likely to collect lint from sheets?
    a. light   c. silk
    b. dark   d. satin _____

23. Who is responsible for instructing the client how to get comfortable on the facial bed?
    a. client   c. manager
    b. receptionist   d. esthetician _____

24. What aspect of services is affected by the considerations of efficiency and laundry costs?
    a. product application
    b. massage technique
    c. draping
    d. hot-towel temperature
    _____

25. When in the process of draping the hair do you place the towel on the headrest?
    a. at any time throughout the process
    b. whenever the client specifically requests you to do so
    c. at the beginning of the process
    d. at the end of the process
    _____

26. What service should you recommend that all clients receive once a month?
    a. facial
    b. Botox® injection
    c. Proactiv® treatment
    d. acupuncture
    _____

27. What step can be dropped when a client is receiving a mini-facial instead of a basic facial?
    a. moisturizer
    b. extractions
    c. product application
    d. draping
    _____

28. What is true of home care?
    a. it is probably the least important factor in successful skin care
    b. it is probably the most important factor in successful skin care
    c. home care has no impact whatsoever on overall skin care
    d. very few clients perform any type of home care on their skin
    _____

29. What should you do for about 15 minutes after the first treatment with a new client?
    a. demonstrate high-priced products
    b. explain why tips affect your income
    c. explain proper home care
    d. perform a client consultation
    _____

30. What is true of a mini-facial?
    a. it has fewer steps than a basic facial
    b. it has more steps than a basic facial
    c. it is the same as a basic facial
    d. it has no treatment benefits
    _____

31. What is the approximate length of a full, basic facial?
    a. 10 minutes
    b. 25 minutes
    c. 45 minutes
    d. 60 minutes
    _____

32. What skin type is associated with the treatment goal of stimulating sebum production?
    a. oily skin
    c. dry skin
    b. couperose skin
    d. damaged skin   ____

33. What type of enzyme peel should you use to exfoliate dry skin?
    a. gentle
    b. medium
    c. harsh
    d. enzyme peels should not be used on dry skin   ____

34. What is **NOT** a recommended treatment for dry skin?
    a. moisturizing cream with an oil base
    b. antioxidants
    c. sunscreen finish
    d. harsh exfoliation   ____

35. What can be caused by exposure to extreme climates, extreme weight loss, and physiological disease?
    a. hypopigmentation
    c. couperose skin
    b. accelerated skin aging
    d. albinism   ____

36. What do facial treatments offer in addition to relaxation?
    a. changes in skin type
    c. weight loss
    b. improving the skin's health
    d. stimulated hair growth   ____

37. What is true of facial treatments?
    a. they are the core treatments that estheticians perform
    b. they are minor elements of the services performed by estheticians
    c. only clients with damaged skin truly benefit from facial treatments
    d. clients with damaged skin are beyond the help of facial treatments   ____

38. What is a facial?
    a. professional service designed to improve and rejuvenate the skin
    b. application of makeup to make the client's face more attractive
    c. medical procedure involving the use of injected chemicals
    d. surgical procedure more commonly known as a face lift   ____

39. Where are corrective treatments the focus?
    a. nail salons
    c. medical offices
    b. beauty salon
    d. day spas   ____

40. Who can issue prescriptions?
    a. receptionists
    c. estheticians
    b. physicians
    d. salon managers _____

41. How often should you attend an esthetics class or conference in order to improve your potential career success?
    a. at least once a month
    b. at least once a year
    c. every few years
    d. never, because classes and conferences are only for beginners _____

42. What can you help clients do by speaking to them in a quiet and professional manner?
    a. believe everything you say
    c. relax
    b. take all of your advice
    d. sleep _____

43. What is a good description of the way you should work with clients?
    a. fast and aggressively
    c. loudly and slowly
    b. quietly and efficiently
    d. casually and haphazardly _____

44. What is **NOT** among the reasons why you should remove rings, bracelets, and other jewelry before performing services?
    a. your nice jewelry will make clients jealous
    b. jewelry might injure the client
    c. jewelry might cause a distraction during the service
    d. jewelry might inhibit your movements during the service _____

45. What is the approximate length of a mini-facial?
    a. five minutes
    c. 20 minutes
    b. 10 minutes
    d. 30 minutes _____

46. What should you do after cleansing the client's skin?
    a. show the client where to change into a robe for the service
    b. complete a thorough skin analysis with a magnifying lamp
    c. perform a client consultation to identify which services to perform
    d. get the client comfortable on the treatment table _____

47. When during the facial procedure should you perform the client consultation?
    a. at the beginning
    c. at the end
    b. in the middle
    d. anytime _____

48. When during the facial procedure should you apply moisturizer and/or sunscreen?
    a. at the beginning
    b. in the middle
    c. at the end
    d. anytime
    ____

49. What is true of skin irritation?
    a. it is a contraindication for a facial
    b. it is always caused by an allergic reaction
    c. it can quickly be eliminated by scrubbing the area with soap and water
    d. it is most commonly seen in people with oily skin
    ____

50. When should you apply warm towels?
    a. before the dry skin analysis
    b. during the dry skin analysis
    c. after the dry skin analysis
    d. at the end of the facial treatment
    ____

51. Who should rinse and flush the client's eyes if product gets into the eyes?
    a. client
    b. physician
    c. esthetician
    d. supervisor
    ____

52. What type of cleanser is difficult to quickly and efficiently remove?
    a. milky
    b. foaming
    c. powdered
    d. liquid
    ____

53. When is exfoliation most effective?
    a. before cleansing
    b. during cleansing
    c. after cleansing
    d. instead of cleansing
    ____

54. What is **NOT** a common result of extreme weight loss?
    a. loss of muscle tone
    b. lined skin
    c. sagging skin
    d. abnormal hair growth
    ____

55. What is **NOT** a beneficial treatment for mature skin?
    a. UV lamp treatment
    b. deep-penetrating serum
    c. firming products
    d. massage
    ____

56. What is **NOT** a beneficial treatment for sensitive skin?
    a. freeze-dried collagen masks
    b. gentle cleansers
    c. harsh cleansers
    d. minimal steam
    ____

57. What are considered vasoconstricting?
    a. hot towels   c. steam treatments
    b. cold towels   d. paraffin masks   _____

58. What is **NOT** contraindicated for sensitive skin?
    a. gentle cleansers   c. hot steam or towels
    b. microdermabrasion   d. vigorous massage   _____

59. What is desincrustation?
    a. process of removing the "crust" that gathers around the eyes
       during sleep
    b. process used to soften oil and comedones in follicles
    c. another name for extractions
    d. another name for exfoliation   _____

60. What is folliculitis?
    a. excessive hair around the face
    b. goose bumps
    c. abnormally low number of hair follicles
    d. inflammation of the hair follicles   _____

61. What is the common name for pseudofolliculitis?
    a. goose bumps   c. wind burn
    b. razor bumps   d. sunburn   _____

62. What causes pseudofolliculitis?
    a. use of hair dye   c. use of Rogaine®
    b. improper shaving   d. poor sleep habits   _____

63. What is a use for cool towels?
    a. preventing folliculitis   c. calming sensitive skin
    b. preventing pseudofolliculitis   d. stimulating sensitive skin _____

64. What skin type benefits from light, water-based products?
    a. couperose skin   c. damaged skin
    b. oily skin   d. mature skin   _____

65. Why should comedogenic products be avoided for clients with acne?
    a. these products are typically water-based
    b. clients with acne experience pain from comedogenic products
    c. clients with acne bleed easily after exposure to comedogenic
       products
    d. these products tend to aggravate or produce acne symptoms _____

CHAPTER 16—FACIAL MASSAGE

1. What action should you **NOT** use on the center of the neck?
   a. pressing down
   b. stroking gently
   c. applying lotion
   d. touching _____

2. What part of the body should you avoid tapping because tapping in that area will feel unpleasant to the client?
   a. forehead
   b. cheeks
   c. neck
   d. jawbone _____

3. What is feathering?
   a. use of feathers for soft touching during a massage
   b. use of quick, bird-like movements during a massage
   c. term for the slowing-down movements at the end of a massage
   d. practice of resting a client on a feather pillow during a massage _____

4. What is true about the décolleté?
   a. that is where you end your massage procedure
   b. this area of the body should be avoided during massage
   c. this is the single most important area during a massage
   d. that is where you begin your massage procedure _____

5. How many milliliters of product should you use on the facial area?
   a. five
   b. 10
   c. 15
   d. 25 _____

6. What is acupressure?
   a. use of needles to stimulate parts of the body
   b. Oriental technique of applying pressure to specific body points
   c. use of measuring tools to ensure precise massage movements
   d. use of a blood-pressure gauge during massage to monitor health _____

7. What is chucking?
   a. application of pressure to specific points of the body
   b. light, continuous stroking movement applied with fingers
   c. deep rubbing movement requiring pressure on the skin
   d. grasping flesh in one hand while the other hand holds the limb _____

8. Why is the Dr. Jacquet movement beneficial to oily skin?
   a. it presses sebum deeper into the follicles, away from the surface
   b. it helps move sebum out of the follicles and up to the skin's surface
   c. the friction of the movement normalizes the skin's pH
   d. it causes the body to stop producing sebum   _____

9. What is effleurage?
   a. use of needles on pressure points
   b. movement involving grasping flesh firmly with one hand
   c. light, continuous stroking movement
   d. deep rubbing movement   _____

10. What is friction?
    a. light, continuous stroking movement
    b. deep rubbing movement
    c. movement involving grasping flesh firmly with one hand
    d. use of needles on pressure points   _____

11. What is **NOT** a variation of friction?
    a. chucking   c. wringing
    b. rolling   d. effleurage   _____

12. What is fulling?
    a. form of petrissage   c. variation of acupressure
    b. form of effleurage   d. variation of shiatsu   _____

13. What is hacking?
    a. deep rubbing movement requiring pressure on the skin
    b. light, continuous stroking movement applied with fingers
    c. movement involving grasping flesh firmly with one hand
    d. chopping movement performed with the edges of the hands   _____

14. What is a characteristic of manual lymph drainage?
    a. aggressive, irregular pressure
    b. gentle, rhythmic pressure
    c. strong chopping motions
    d. hard kneading movements   _____

15. What is the term for the manual or mechanical manipulation of the body by using movements to increase metabolism and circulation, among other effects?
    a. massage   c. physical therapy
    b. acupuncture   d. reconditioning   _____

16. What improves overall metabolism and activates sluggish skin?
    a. caffeine
    b. massage
    c. sun exposure
    d. sugar
    _____

17. What should be performed for approximately 10 to 15 minutes during a facial?
    a. extractions
    b. facial massage
    c. steaming
    d. manicure/pedicure
    _____

18. What must estheticians be in order to perform deep tissue work?
    a. licensed massage therapists (LMTs)
    b. emergency medical technicians (EMTs)
    c. licensed medical technicians (LMTs)
    d. emergency massage technicians (EMTs)
    _____

19. Where should massage movements begin?
    a. insertion
    b. origin
    c. joint
    d. any point along the muscle   _____

20. What do inflamed acne, open lesions, and sunburn have in common?
    a. clients with these conditions are badly in need of massage
    b. massage is contraindicated for clients with these conditions
    c. clients with these conditions should only receive gentle massage
    d. clients with these conditions should only receive vigorous massage
    _____

21. When should you avoid vigorous massage?
    a. when you are too tired to perform vigorous massage
    b. when you don't feel a client deserves vigorous massage
    c. when a client has arthritis or other pain
    d. when a client has oily skin
    _____

22. When should you advise a client with reservations about facial massage to speak with a physician?
    a. after the first massage session
    b. before performing massage
    c. after a month of regular massage
    d. after a year of regular massage
    _____

23. What type of movements are used in petrissage?
    a. kneading
    b. chopping
    c. poking
    d. tapping
    _____

24. Where do you apply pressure when performing reflexology?
    a. hands   c. legs
    b. shoulders   d. feet   ____

25. What is rolling?
    a. pressing and twisting tissues using a back-and-forth movement
    b. pressing but not twisting tissues
    c. twisting but not pressing tissues
    d. pressing and twisting tissues using a special tool similar to a rolling pin   ____

26. What is **NOT** a type of movement characteristic of tapotement?
    a. tapping   c. kneading
    b. slapping   d. hacking   ____

27. What is a form of acupressure?
    a. effleurage   c. Dr. Jacquet movement
    b. petrissage   d. shiatsu   ____

28. What part of the esthetician's body must be kept flexible during slapping to ensure that the palms come into proper contact with the body?
    a. wrists   c. shoulders
    b. elbows   d. hips   ____

29. What type of movements are used in vibration?
    a. rapid striking   c. slow striking
    b. rapid shaking   d. slow shaking   ____

30. When do the body's reflex receptors increase blood and lymph flow, resulting in a state of relaxation?
    a. when touch is sensed by the body
    b. when heat is sensed by the body
    c. when cold is sensed by the body
    d. when moisture is sensed by the body   ____

31. What does the central nervous system trigger when affected by massage?
    a. rapid heartbeat   c. stress
    b. "fight-or-flight" reaction   d. relaxation   ____

32. To whom should you refer a client who wants a full body massage?
    a. physical therapist   c. licensed massage therapist
    b. nurse practitioner   d. chiropractor   ____

33. What information can be found by referring to licensing regulations?
    a. product ingredients
    c. scope of practice
    b. pricing scales
    d. customer demographics ____

34. What should you do during effleurage in order to avoid scratching the client?
    a. avoid using lotions that might make the work surface slippery
    b. avoid using the ends of your fingertips
    c. avoid working in a warmth that might induce client perspiration
    d. wear thick gloves to ensure your skin doesn't touch the client's skin ____

35. What is true of tapotement?
    a. it is the most stimulating form of massage
    b. it is the least stimulating form of massage
    c. it is not a stimulating form of massage
    d. only licensed massage technicians can perform tapotement ____

36. How long should vibration be used on any one spot of the body?
    a. no more than a few seconds
    b. no more than a minute
    c. no more than 10 minutes
    d. no more than 20 minutes ____

37. What is true of the left and right sides of the areas being massaged?
    a. left side should receive more vigorous massage
    b. right side should receive more vigorous massage
    c. both sides of the body should be massaged simultaneously
    d. movements should be duplicated on both the right and left sides ____

38. What everyday movement is somewhat similar to the Dr. Jacquet movement?
    a. squeezing the peel of an orange to make juice spray out
    b. plucking seeds from a watermelon
    c. peeling an apple
    d. cracking open a walnut ____

39. Why should the Dr. Jacquet movement be avoided on areas of the skin that are infected or irritated?
    a. client will experience piercing pain in those areas
    b. client will experience sudden bleeding in those areas
    c. too much pressure will rupture follicle walls
    d. will cause an infection or irritation to rapidly spread all over the body _____

40. What type of movements are appropriate when massaging the area of beard growth on male clients?
    a. downward   c. sideways
    b. upward   d. diagonal   _____

CHAPTER 17—FACIAL MACHINES

1. How does dehydrated skin appear under a Wood's Lamp?
   a. light violet/purple
   b. deep crimson/red
   c. light turquoise/blue
   d. deep emerald/green ____

2. What is **NOT** one of the colors comedones will assume when viewed under a Wood's Lamp?
   a. yellow
   b. pink
   c. orange
   d. green ____

3. How will hypopigmentation appear under a Wood's Lamp?
   a. red-purple or beige-brown
   b. blue-white or yellow-green
   c. orange-yellow or gray-black
   d. black-red or brown-gray ____

4. What machine helps address excess cell buildup, excess dirt, and excess oil?
   a. steamer
   b. rotary brush
   c. galvanic current
   d. electric mitts ____

5. When in the rotary-brush procedure should you lightly cleanse the client's skin?
   a. before the service
   b. halfway through the service
   c. after the service
   d. throughout the entire service ____

6. How long should a rotary brush be used on each area during each of your three passes?
   a. three to five seconds
   b. seven to 10 seconds
   c. 12 to 15 seconds
   d. 17 to 20 seconds ____

7. How often should you remove brushes from the rotary brush machine, wash them with soap and water, and immerse them in disinfectant per manufacturer recommendations?
   a. once per day
   b. once per week
   c. after every client
   d. after every few clients ____

8. Why should you avoid using tap water in steamers?
   a. calcium buildups in tap water necessitate extra cleaning
   b. mineral deposits in tap water give steam an unpleasant odor
   c. calcium and mineral deposits in tap water might damage machinery
   d. tap water is not thick enough to be used with a steamer ____

9. What is the ordinary steam-treatment time during a facial?
   a. between eight and 10 minutes
   b. between 10 and 20 minutes
   c. between 30 and 35 minutes
   d. about one hour   ____

10. What function does the rotary brush perform?
    a. aggressive extraction
    b. gentle extraction
    c. light exfoliation and stimulation
    d. heavy exfoliation and stimulation   ____

11. What is sebum transformed into via the chemical reaction of saponification?
    a. lymph   c. oil
    b. soap   d. cold cream   ____

12. What is **NOT** true of sinusoidal current?
    a. it is a smooth, repetitive current
    b. it is an alternating current
    c. it produces heat effects
    d. use on the scalp is contraindicated   ____

13. What is a misting device used for facial treatments?
    a. spray machine   c. high-frequency machine
    b. vacuum machine   d. steamer   ____

14. What is a heat effect that is used for permanent hair removal?
    a. saponification   c. anaphoresis
    b. desincrustation   d. thermolysis   ____

15. What is the purpose of a vacuum machine?
    a. cleaning debris after facial treatments
    b. removing impurities and stimulating circulation
    c. quickly removing makeup before a facial treatment
    d. extracting fine facial hairs left behind after shaving ____

16. What type of light does a Wood's Lamp use?
    a. white light   c. red light
    b. blue light   d. black light   ____

17. When should you ask a client to get a doctor's note?
    a. prior to any facial services
    b. prior to using facial machines
    c. if you have doubts about whether the client can have electrotherapy
    d. if you have doubts about whether the client practices good home care _____

18. When in the process of using electrical devices should you ask clients to remove jewelry?
    a. when you get close to working in the area of the jewelry
    b. only if the jewelry is large and cumbersome
    c. before beginning the procedure
    d. after completing the procedure _____

19. What is forced into tissues during anaphoresis?
    a. positive liquids   c. positive gases
    b. negative liquids   d. negative gases _____

20. What device is used for cataphoresis?
    a. Tesla high-frequency current   c. violet ray
    b. galvanic current   d. steamer _____

21. What is emulsified or liquefied during desincrustation?
    a. sebum and debris   c. oil and water
    b. lymph and debris   d. lymph and water _____

22. What is the term for the use of electronic devices for therapeutic benefits?
    a. electrified therapy   c. electrotherapy
    b. electrolysis   d. electronic therapy _____

23. What is **NOT** true of galvanic current?
    a. it is a constant current
    b. it is a direct current
    c. it produces chemical reactions
    d. it is contraindicated for the face _____

24. What sort of effect is generated by a high-frequency machine?
    a. gentle warming   c. gentle cooling
    b. strong heat   d. strong cold _____

25. What are ions?
    a. atoms or molecules carrying a negative electrical charge
    b. atoms or molecules carrying a positive electrical charge
    c. atoms or molecules carrying any electrical charge
    d. atoms or molecules that cannot carry an electrical charge   _____

26. What is ionization?
    a. process of fortifying a substance with additional ions
    b. process of separating a substance into ions
    c. process of identifying and cataloguing ions
    d. process of merging ions to form a new substance   _____

27. What does iontophoresis create?
    a. acidic reaction that contracts the skin
    b. acidic reaction that relaxes the skin
    c. alkaline reaction that contracts the skin
    d. alkaline reaction that relaxes the skin   _____

28. What term refers to an atomizer designed to apply plant extracts
    and other ingredients to the skin?
    a. botanic sprayer   c. steamer plug
    b. spritzing mister   d. Lucas sprayer   _____

29. What should you do with your steamer once steam is visible?
    a. begin the treatment without any further steps
    b. turn on the second switch (the ozone or vaporizer)
    c. turn off the second switch (the ozone or vaporizer)
    d. turn the device off to prevent it from overheating   _____

30. What should you do with your steamer after each use?
    a. turn it off for one hour
    b. clean and disinfect it
    c. top off the water in the reservoir
    d. add bleach to the water in the reservoir to prevent
       bacterial growth   _____

31. What is **NOT** true about essential oils as they relate to the
    process of using a steamer?
    a. they should be placed in a wick-like apparatus near the
       nozzle
    b. they should be deposited directly into the steamer's water
       supply
    c. essential oils should be treated the same way as herbs
    d. essential oils can be a helpful addition to a steam treatment   _____

32. What treatment can be replaced with the use of a vacuum machine?
    a. product application
    b. steam treatment
    c. massage
    d. extractions
    _____

33. What purpose does a piece of cotton serve when inserted into the hand piece of a vacuum machine?
    a. temperature regulation
    b. speed regulation
    c. filtration
    d. disinfection
    _____

34. What can you avoid by lifting your finger off the hold of a vacuum machine before lifting the device off the face?
    a. infecting the skin
    b. burning the skin
    c. cutting the skin
    d. pulling the skin
    _____

35. What sort of storage is appropriate for vacuum-machine tips?
    a. heated
    b. refrigerated
    c. covered container
    d. uncovered container
    _____

36. What type of skin is helped by desincrustation because the process helps soften and relax the debris in follicles?
    a. normal
    b. mature
    c. dry
    d. oily
    _____

37. Where is an appropriate place to warm cotton pads and products?
    a. microwave
    b. hot plate
    c. paraffin wax heater
    d. towel warmer
    _____

38. How often should you clean the inside of the hot-towel cabinet with a topical disinfectant?
    a. once per day
    b. once per week
    c. once every hour
    d. after each client session
    _____

39. What should you do to the water catchment tray underneath the hot-towel cabinet's caddy on a daily basis?
    a. simply wipe it down with a paper towel
    b. rinse it with water and let it air dry
    c. empty, clean, and disinfect it
    d. discard and replace it
    _____

40. What is the most common magnification for magnifying lamps, measured in diopters?
    a. five
    b. 10
    c. 15
    d. 20
    _____

41. What is **NOT** a common cause of eyestrain?
    a. steam in the treatment room
    b. improper illumination
    c. distortion on the magnifying lamp
    d. insufficient illumination _____

42. What is sometimes known as a "loupe"?
    a. tweezers   c. magnifying lamp
    b. Wood's Lamp   d. steamer _____

43. When should you loosen the adjustment knobs on your
    magnifying lamp?
    a. at the start of every day   c. never
    b. at the end of every day   d. whenever you move the arms _____

44. What should you **AVOID** using on the lens of your magnifying
    lamp?
    a. lens tissue   c. paper products
    b. lens-cleaning fluid   d. soft cloth _____

45. How will a thick corneum layer appear under a Wood's Lamp?
    a. red blotches   c. white fluorescence
    b. black blotches   d. blue fluorescence _____

CHAPTER 18—HAIR REMOVAL

1. What is the third stage of hair growth?
   a. anagen
   b. catagen
   c. latent
   d. telogen
   ____

2. How does thermolysis destroy hair follicles?
   a. shattering them with sound
   b. clogging them with sebum
   c. burning them with heat
   d. sealing them with light
   ____

3. What is another name for threading?
   a. stitching
   b. attaching
   c. weaving
   d. banding
   ____

4. What is trichology?
   a. scientific study of hair-removal techniques
   b. scientific study of hair and its diseases
   c. technical term for mechanically removing hair
   d. technical term for artificially coloring hair
   ____

5. What is vellus hair?
   a. fine, soft, downy hair
   b. short, coarse, shaved hair
   c. heavy, thick, strong hair
   d. hair found on the back and shoulders
   ____

6. What is oily skin a contraindication for?
   a. hair removal
   b. acne treatments
   c. waxing
   d. extractions
   ____

7. What is **NOT** a contraindication for facial waxing?
   a. recent cosmetic surgery
   b. recent reconstructive surgery
   c. recent laser treatments
   d. recent steam treatments
   ____

8. How long must hair be in order to remove it with waxing?
   a. 1/4-inch
   b. 1/2-inch
   c. 3/4-inch
   d. 2/3-inch
   ____

9. What should clients avoid for at least 24 to 48 hours after waxing?
   a. moisture
   b. exercise
   c. salty foods
   d. excessive heat
   ____

10. What can lead to the production of new terminal hairs?
    a. removing fine (vellus) hair on areas not covered by terminal hairs
    b. applying heat to areas not covered by terminal hairs
    c. applying moisture to areas not covered by terminal hairs
    d. conditioning fine (vellus) hairs on areas not covered by terminal hairs ____

11. What happens to lanugo hair shortly after birth?
    a. replaced exclusively by vellus hairs
    b. replaced either by vellus hairs or by terminal hairs
    c. replaced exclusively by terminal hairs
    d. falls off, leaving those parts of the skin perfectly smooth ____

12. When happens during puberty?
    a. lanugo hairs are lost by the body
    b. follicles switch from producing vellus hairs to terminal hairs
    c. follicles switch from producing terminal hairs to vellus hairs
    d. lanugo hairs emerge on the body ____

13. What is the acronym ACT used to help estheticians remember?
    a. procedural steps for a basic facial
    b. safety steps for mechanical hair removal
    c. layers of the skin from outermost to innermost
    d. stages of hair growth ____

14. What is anagen?
    a. first stage of hair growth
    b. second stage of hair growth
    c. third stage of hair growth
    d. fourth stage of hair growth ____

15. What describes the arrector pili muscle?
    a. muscle that moves the nostrils
    b. muscle that moves the lips
    c. appendage of the hair follicle
    d. appendage of the sweat glands ____

16. What is infected inflammation of the hair follicle?
    a. benign follicutosis   c. tinea follicutosis
    b. barbae folliculitis   d. acute folliculastis ____

17. What is the second stage of hair growth?
    a. catagen   c. latent
    b. anagen   d. telogen ____

18. What is the function of a depilatory?
    a. permanently removing superfluous hair by extracting the root
    b. temporarily removing superfluous hair by extracting the root
    c. permanently removing superfluous hair by dissolving it at skin level
    d. temporarily removing superfluous hair by dissolving it at skin level   ____

19. What is the removal of hair by means of an electric current that destroys the hair root?
    a. anagen   c. electrolysis
    b. catagen   d. epilation   ____

20. What is removing hair from the follicles via tweezing or waxing?
    a. electrolysis   c. anagen
    b. epilation   d. catagen   ____

21. Where is the hair bulb located?
    a. interior shaft of the follicle
    b. exterior shaft of the follicle
    c. outermost tip of the follicle
    d. base of the follicle   ____

22. What shape does a hair follicle take?
    a. perfect square   c. small sphere
    b. elongated triangle   d. small tube   ____

23. Why is it beneficial that each thread is discarded after use during the threading process?
    a. allows you to charge clients more for additional thread
    b. makes threading more sanitary than waxing
    c. ensures more direct contact than with waxing
    d. reduces the amount of motions in threading   ____

24. What type of skin might benefit from sugaring as an alternative form of epilation?
    a. oily   c. pale
    b. sensitive   d. dark   ____

25. What direction is product applied during the hand method of sugaring?
    a. toward the center of the torso
    b. away from the center of the torso
    c. with the hair growth
    d. against the hair growth   ____

26. What direction is product applied during the spatula method of sugaring?
    a. toward the center of the torso
    b. away from the center of the torso
    c. with the hair growth
    d. against the hair growth ____

27. What epilation technique is associated with the dangers of burns severe enough for blisters, failure to remove hair, and the removal of actual skin?
    a. waxing
    b. threading
    c. spatula-method sugaring
    d. hand-method sugaring ____

28. What is **NOT** a form in which hard waxes are available?
    a. blocks
    b. pellets
    c. beads
    d. strips ____

29. What is true of soft wax?
    a. has a lower melting point than hard wax
    b. has a higher melting point than hard wax
    c. available only in tins
    d. must always be applied thickly ____

30. What is true of stainless steel slant-tipped tweezers?
    a. they are best for general tweezing
    b. they are best for removing ingrown hairs
    c. they will corrode when disinfected in solution
    d. they break down easily ____

31. What is pellon used to make?
    a. dermal fillers
    b. paraffin masks
    c. enzyme peel ingredients
    d. wax strips ____

32. What is the shape of the hair papilla?
    a. box
    b. tube
    c. cone
    d. triangle ____

33. What function does the hair root perform?
    a. infusing color into the hair
    b. connecting hair to the bones
    c. feeding nutrients to the hair
    d. anchoring the hair to the skin cells ____

34. What is hirsutism?
    a. outgrowths of downy hair on body parts usually bearing terminal hair
    b. outgrowths of ingrown downy hairs causing skin irritation
    c. unusual hair loss on body parts normally bearing downy hair
    d. unusual hair growth on body parts normally bearing downy hair ____

35. What is the term for excessive hair growth where hair does not normally grow?
    a. hypertrichosis   c. epilation
    b. hypopigmentation   d. lanugo   ____

36. What does the acronym IPL stand for?
    a. intermittent phased light
    b. intermediate power light
    c. intense pulsed light
    d. integumentary patterned lesions   ____

37. When in life does the human body grow lanugo hair?
    a. old age   c. puberty
    b. middle age   d. gestation   ____

38. What is **NOT** true of laser hair removal?
    a. it is a type of photoepilation
    b. it involves pulsing a laser on skin
    c. hair removed by this method tends to grow back quickly
    d. several wavelengths are used at a time   ____

39. What does photoepilation use to remove hair?
    a. galvanic current and shaving
    b. IPL and laser hair removal
    c. IPL and shaving
    d. galvanic current and laser hair removal   ____

40. What is **NOT** contained within the pilosebaceous unit?
    a. hair root   c. dermal papilla
    b. bulb   d. sebaceous gland   ____

41. What is an ancient method of hair removal?
    a. sweetening   c. sharpening
    b. shortening   d. sugaring   ____

42. How long does a hair located on the scalp grow each month, on average?
    a. one-half inch   c. two inches
    b. one inch   d. three inches   ____

43. When does the latent phase of hair growth occur?
    a. between catagen and telogen
    b. between anagen and catagen
    c. after anagen and before telogen
    d. after telogen and before anagen   ____

44. What is considered to be the only true method of permanent hair removal?
    a. IPL   c. depilation
    b. laser hair removal   d. electrolysis   ____

45. What hair-removal procedure is performed by inserting small needles into the hair follicles?
    a. sugaring   c. threading
    b. electrolysis   d. waxing   ____

46. What effect does galvanic electrolysis have?
    a. sealing the hair follicle shut through severe burning
    b. quickly yanking the entire hair shaft out by the root
    c. chemical alteration of the skin pH in the area near the follicle
    d. chemical decomposition of the hair follicle   ____

47. What is **NOT** true of shaving?
    a. it can irritate the skin
    b. it is a daily ritual for many men
    c. it is a daily ritual for many women
    d. it permanently removes hair   ____

48. What can be corrected by changing the direction of shaving?
    a. prevalence of ingrown hairs   c. speed of hair growth
    b. need for frequent shaving   d. density of hair growth   ____

49. For what type of skin is tweezing often a better alternative to shaving?
    a. oily   c. normal
    b. dry   d. sensitive   ____

CHAPTER 19—ADVANCED TOPICS AND TREATMENTS

1. What effect does sclerotherapy have on varicose veins?
    a. minimizes them
    b. enlarges them
    c. destroys them
    d. reroutes them
    ____

2. What parts of the face are affected by the procedure transconjuctival blepharoplasty?
    a. nostrils
    b. lower lips
    c. cheeks
    d. lower eyelids
    ____

3. What is a TCA peel used for?
    a. lightening highly pigmented skin
    b. darkening lightly pigmented skin
    c. diminishing sun damage and wrinkles
    d. preventing collagen and elastin production
    ____

4. What happens to our cell renewal factor (CRF) as we age?
    a. becomes more intense
    b. goes away completely
    c. speeds up
    d. slows down
    ____

5. What is a procedure that only physicians can administer?
    a. deep peels
    b. chemical peels
    c. clay masks
    d. paraffin masks
    ____

6. What is an acceptable pH level for salon peels based on professional recommendations and, in most states, legal restrictions?
    a. 1.5 or higher
    b. 2.0 or higher
    c. 2.5 or higher
    d. 3.0 or higher
    ____

7. What is true of open sores and suspicious lesions?
    a. they have no bearing on the choice to perform chemical exfoliation
    b. their presence requires extra care during chemical exfoliation
    c. these conditions sometimes contraindicate chemical exfoliation
    d. these conditions always contraindicate chemical exfoliation
    ____

8. What is **NOT** something that clients should be advised to avoid for at least 24 to 48 hours in advance of a chemical exfoliation procedure?
    a. soap-and-water cleansing
    b. sun exposure
    c. benzoyl peroxide applications
    d. waxing
    ____

9. A person with what condition would benefit more from microdermabrasion than other forms of exfoliation?
   a. oily skin
   b. dry skin
   c. inability to tolerate alkalis
   d. inability to tolerate acids _____

10. What treatment can have the effects of hyperpigmentation, hypopigmentation, and/or sensitivity if administered improperly?
   a. paraffin masks   c. extraction
   b. clay masks   d. microdermabrasion _____

11. What does an abdominoplasty involve?
   a. removing excess fat and loose skin from the abdomen
   b. exfoliating the skin along the abdomen
   c. removing hair along the abdomen
   d. massaging the abdominal muscles to stimulate muscle growth _____

12. What spa treatment is based on the concept of three doshas?
   a. foot reflexology   c. Ayurvedic treatments
   b. stone massage   d. Reiki _____

13. What are commonly used in balneotherapy body treatments?
   a. powerful water jets   c. hot stones
   b. Dead Sea salts   d. cold stones _____

14. What is **NOT** a benefit of body scrubs?
   a. detoxifying the body   c. exfoliation
   b. increasing circulation   d. hydration _____

15. What **PRIMARILY** determines the effect of a body wrap?
   a. material used to wrap the client
   b. type of product used
   c. length of time the client is wrapped
   d. positioning of the client while wrapped _____

16. What is Botox®?
   a. highly acidic cream
   b. neuromuscular-blocking serum
   c. type of acne medication
   d. surgical procedure for removing fat from the abdomen _____

17. What is a characteristic of the people whose hips are **MOST** likely to contain cellulite?
   a. they have oily skin   c. they are overweight
   b. they have dry skin   d. they are underweight _____

18. What is **NOT** something that dermal fillers are used to fill?
    a. facial imperfections   c. lines
    b. pores   d. wrinkles   ____

19. What is mammoplasty?
    a. abdominal surgery   c. facial surgery
    b. breast surgery   d. a type of liposuction   ____

20. What does the esthetician use to move congestion, water, and waste in the lymphatic vessels out of the body when performing MLD?
    a. massage   c. galvanic current
    b. microcurrent   d. reiki   ____

21. What device mimics the body's natural electrical energy to reeducate and tone facial muscles?
    a. laser machine   c. microcurrent machine
    b. steamer   d. microdermabrasion machine   ____

22. What is a form of mechanical exfoliation?
    a. mammoplasty   c. manual lymph drainage
    b. microdermabrasion   d. microcurrent   ____

23. What type of treatments does the term "nonablative" refer to?
    a. acne   c. cellulite
    b. wrinkle   d. hypopigmentation   ____

24. What treatments employ the use of phenol (carbolic acid)?
    a. peels   c. exfoliations
    b. extractions   d. massages   ____

25. What is **NOT** true of reconstructive surgery?
    a. it restores a bodily function
    b. it is performed on accident survivors
    c. it is performed on those with congenital defects
    d. it is a form of cosmetic surgery   ____

26. What is a rhytidectomy?
    a. tummy tuck   c. face lift
    b. breast enhancement   d. nose job   ____

27. What is the technical term for nose surgery that makes a nose smaller or changes its appearance?
    a. rhinoplasty   c. blepharoplasty
    b. rhytidectomy   d. proboscistomy   ____

28. What condition does endermology treat?
    a. acne
    b. albinism
    c. sensitive skin
    d. cellulite
    ____

29. What is the technical term for an eye lift?
    a. rhinoplasty
    b. blepharoplasty
    c. oculoplasty
    d. hippoplasty
    ____

30. What is the term for spa treatments that use water?
    a. aquatherapy
    b. hydrotherapy
    c. liquid therapy
    d. immersion therapy
    ____

31. What purpose to injectable fillers serve?
    a. pain relief
    b. stress relief
    c. skin darkening
    d. skin plumping
    ____

32. What is the term for the application of light rays to the skin for the treatment of wrinkles, capillaries, pigmentation, and hair removal?
    a. sclerotherapy
    b. endotherapy
    c. ultrasonic therapy
    d. light therapy
    ____

33. What is a procedure that surgically removes pockets of fat?
    a. liposuction
    b. rhinoplasty
    c. sclerotherapy
    d. laser resurfacing
    ____

34. What tool is used to physically remove tissue down to the dermis during mechanical dermabrasion?
    a. brush
    b. blade
    c. file
    d. sponge
    ____

35. What is **NOT** an ingredient of a Jessner's peel?
    a. citric acid
    b. lactic acid
    c. salicylic acid
    d. resorcinol
    ____

CHAPTER 20—THE WORLD OF MAKEUP

1. What type of light is **BEST** for makeup application?
   a. natural
   b. incandescent
   c. fluorescent
   d. LED
   _____

2. What is one of the factors to consider when choosing colors for a client?
   a. skin type
   b. skin color
   c. skin pH
   d. skin density
   _____

3. What is **NOT** true of the color temperature green?
   a. bright green can downplay red in the skin
   b. it is easy on the eyes
   c. it is flattering to many skin tones
   d. blue-greens are cool
   _____

4. What is true of the color temperature brown?
   a. it is a drab and unflattering color rarely used in makeup
   b. it can be kind to many complexion tones
   c. it is only flattering to dark complexion tones
   d. it is only flattering to pale complexion tones
   _____

5. What is **NOT** true of the beige skin tone?
   a. it is a medium skin tone
   b. it may have pink undertones
   c. it may have yellow undertones
   d. it may have green undertones
   _____

6. What skin tone has creamy or slightly pink undertones?
   a. deep or black
   b. olive or hot
   c. beige or median
   d. ivory to fair
   _____

7. What hue does sallow skin have?
   a. pinkish
   b. reddish
   c. greenish
   d. yellowish
   _____

8. What type of skin would **NOT** be called ruddy?
   a. red skin
   b. wind-burned skin
   c. skin affected by rosacea
   d. skin affected by albinism
   _____

9. What is the complementary color to orange?
   a. blue
   b. red
   c. yellow
   d. green
   _____

10. What is the complementary color to red?
    a. blue   c. green
    b. yellow   d. orange   _____

11. What are the elements of a shade?
    a. pure hue plus black   c. pure hue plus white
    b. pure hue plus gray   d. pure hue plus yellow   _____

12. What are the elements of a tone?
    a. pure hue plus black   c. pure hue plus white
    b. pure hue plus gray   d. pure hue plus yellow   _____

13. What is **NOT** one of the reasons a particular makeup product
    might be more expensive than another product?
    a. higher-quality ingredients   c. larger advertising budget
    b. more elaborate packaging   d. FDA approval   _____

14. What is **NOT** true of primers?
    a. they are liquid or silicone-based formulas
    b. they are designed to go underneath foundations
    c. they are designed to penetrate into the deepest layer of
       the skin
    d. they prepare the skin for makeup and help keep product
       on the skin   _____

15. What type of makeup is considered healthy because it is less
    heavy, more noncomedogenic, and more natural than other types
    of makeup?
    a. chemical   c. mineral
    b. synthetic   d. acrylic   _____

16. Who often prefers liquid foundation over mineral makeup because
    mineral makeup can sometimes tend to be shiny and too drying?
    a. clients with combination skin c. young clients
    b. male clients   d. mature clients   _____

17. What sort of finish does face powder add to the face?
    a. sheer   c. matte
    b. translucent   d. shiny   _____

18. What is **NOT** a form in which cheek color is commonly available?
    a. cream   c. powder
    b. liquid   d. spray   _____

19. What is true of the eyes?
    a. they are the focal point in makeup design
    b. because makeup cannot be applied onto the eyes, they are
       unimportant
    c. the goal of the makeup artist is to downplay the eyes
    d. makeup that accentuates the eyes has been applied improperly   _____

20. What sort of look do liquid or gel eyeliners create, as opposed to
    pencil eyeliners?
    a. more subdued   c. more dramatic
    b. more natural   d. more cheap   _____

21. What are band lashes?
    a. lashes enlarged by infection
    b. patches where lashes are absent
    c. lashes laden with heavy makeup
    d. artificial lashes on a strip   _____

22. What is cake makeup used for?
    a. light coverage
    b. heavy coverage
    c. giving the eyes a dramatic look
    d. downplaying the appearance of the eyes   _____

23. What is the relationship on the color wheel between
    complementary colors?
    a. they are next to each other
    b. they are one color removed from each other
    c. they are two colors removed from each other
    d. they are opposite each other   _____

24. What are concealers used to cover?
    a. poorly applied makeup
    b. blemishes and discoloration
    c. a client's natural skin color
    d. unwanted hair growth   _____

25. What undertones do cool colors have?
    a. red   c. green
    b. yellow   d. blue   _____

26. What is attached to a client in the procedure called eye tabbing?
    a. band lashes   c. eye shadow
    b. mascara   d. individual lashes   _____

27. What is another name for foundation?
    a. mascara
    c. base makeup
    b. lip liner
    d. concealer
    _____

28. What is greasepaint typically used for?
    a. glamorous evening look
    c. theatrical purposes
    b. casual daytime look
    d. pharmaceutical purposes
    _____

29. What is the term that means "nonshiny or dull"?
    a. translucent
    c. prismatic
    b. iridescent
    d. matte
    _____

30. What is **NOT** an effect mascara has on eyelashes?
    a. darkens
    c. defines
    b. thickens
    d. elongates
    _____

31. What is a large, soft brush used for blending and applying powder or blush?
    a. blush brush
    c. concealer brush
    b. powder brush
    d. kabuki brush
    _____

32. What is a short brush with dense bristles for powder or blush?
    a. angle brow brush
    c. lash and brow brush
    b. lip brush
    d. kabuki brush
    _____

33. What is a blush brush?
    a. smaller version of the powder brush
    b. larger version of the powder brush
    c. smaller version of the kabuki brush
    d. larger version of the kabuki brush
    _____

34. What can you do to prevent brush bristles to dry in the shape they are left in while wet?
    a. avoid washing brushes and simply discard them when dirtied
    b. avoid using moisture, including water, to wash brushes
    c. reshape the wet bristles and lay the brush flat to dry
    d. any shape the bristles dry into after cleaning is acceptable
    _____

35. What is the purpose of using a neck strip?
    a. to keep the cape clean from one client to the next
    b. to enhance the moisturizer you place on the client's neck
    c. to give you a surface for wiping your hands during makeup application
    d. to give you a surface to wipe excess makeup off brushes
    _____

36. What is the term for fundamental colors that cannot be obtained from a mixture?
   a. primary colors
   b. secondary colors
   c. tertiary colors
   d. lakes
   _____

37. What is the term for colors obtained by mixing equal parts of two primary colors?
   a. secondary colors
   b. tertiary colors
   c. derivative colors
   d. mixed colors
   _____

38. What is the term for colors that are formed by mixing equal amounts of a secondary color and its neighboring primary color?
   a. complementary colors
   b. derivative colors
   c. coordinating colors
   d. tertiary colors
   _____

39. What undertones do warm colors have?
   a. blue
   b. red
   c. green
   d. yellow
   _____

40. What are the three primary colors?
   a. green, orange, purple
   b. green, yellow, orange
   c. white, black, gray
   d. red, blue, yellow
   _____

41. What color is created when blue and yellow are mixed together?
   a. purple
   b. green
   c. orange
   d. brown
   _____

42. What color is created when red and yellow are mixed together?
   a. green
   b. orange
   c. purple
   d. brown
   _____

43. What is an example of a tertiary color?
   a. blue
   b. white
   c. purple
   d. blue-violet
   _____

44. What is hue?
   a. specific density of a color
   b. malleability of a color
   c. distinct characteristic of a color
   d. temperature of a color
   _____

45. What are the elements of a tint?
   a. pure hue plus black
   b. pure hue plus gray
   c. pure hue plus white
   d. pure hue plus yellow
   _____

Part 5: Business Skills

CHAPTER 21—CAREER PLANNING

1. When should you start keeping careful track of what you are spending, if you have not already done so?
   a. when you start earning a salary   c. when you reach age 21
   b. when you've had a job for a year   d. when you reach age 25   ____

2. What is **NOT** an indication that you might benefit from professional financial advice?
   a. when you have difficulty managing money
   b. when you feel unsure about how to handle your bank account
   c. when you feel unsure about how to handle your retirement
   d. when you realize you have money left over after paying your bills   ____

3. What is **NOT** something for which you will be responsible if you accept employment as an independent contractor?
   a. insurance   c. compliance with laws
   b. taxes   d. building maintenance fees   ____

4. What amount is used by clients to calculate tips?
   a. total service ticket
   b. amount charged for retail products
   c. price of the basic facial
   d. price of the basic facial plus any add-ons   ____

5. What statement about tips is correct?
   a. all salons allow estheticians to accept tips
   b. only full-time employees may accept tips
   c. tips are considered part of your taxable income
   d. the standard tip is about 10 to 12 percent   ____

6. When should you answer the questions on a test for which you are sure of the answers?
   a. after completing the most difficult questions
   b. when you need a break from more difficult questions
   c. at the beginning, so you save time for difficult questions
   d. you should answer all questions in the order in which they appear on the test   ____

7. What should you do when you come across a difficult question on a test?
   a. work through it and put down an answer before moving on
   b. skip it and come back to it later
   c. skip it altogether, leaving the answer blank
   d. guess at the answer and move on _____

8. What is an advantage of booth rental over other business structures?
   a. significantly lower expenses
   b. shared risk with a partner
   c. capital provided by investors
   d. ownership of the salon building _____

9. What is a destination spa?
   a. spa area of a franchise salon
   b. all-inclusive retreat
   c. spa area of a medical practice
   d. local day spa _____

10. What do full-service salons typically offer?
    a. medical aesthetic procedures
    b. nutrition counseling
    c. a total beauty experience
    d. guest rooms for an extended stay _____

11. What is a focus of treatment at wellness spas?
    a. optimal health maintenance   c. cosmetic surgery
    b. surgical procedures   d. chemical skin treatments _____

12. What is **NOT** a location where one might expect to find a medical spa?
    a. dermatology office   c. hospital
    b. laser center   d. country club _____

13. What form of compensation specifies a certain amount of pay based on a flat or hourly rate?
    a. commission   c. quota
    b. gratuity   d. salary _____

14. What behavior characterizes a test-wise student?
    a. cramming the day before a test
    b. cheating without getting caught
    c. practicing good study habits
    d. answering all questions quickly _____

15. What are transferable skills?
    a. skills you are able to quickly teach to co-workers
    b. skills mastered at one job that are applicable to a new position
    c. skills that you must learn in order to succeed at a specific salon
    d. skills learned in the salon that can also be applied at home _____

16. Why is it important to be an active student?
    a. to become friends with your teacher
    b. to pass the license exam
    c. to make the teacher give you extra credit for classroom involvement
    d. to intimidate other students by showing how assertive you are _____

17. What should you do to prepare yourself for the test?
    a. discard class handouts and focus entirely on the textbook
    b. stay up late studying and get up early to study some more before class
    c. maintain a pessimistic attitude
    d. take effective notes during class _____

18. What should you do to avoid cramming the night before a test?
    a. skip class the day before the test so you can stay home and study
    b. plan your study schedule
    c. study only in the morning
    d. study only when the mood strikes you _____

19. What is commission?
    a. flat-rate form of pay based upon hours worked
    b. percentage-based form of pay related to performance
    c. flat-rate form of pay based upon job description
    d. sliding-scale form of pay based upon experience _____

20. What is the term for the process of reaching logical conclusions by employing logical reasoning?
    a. reductive analysis   c. deductive reasoning
    b. instructive reasoning   d. constructive analysis _____

21. What is **NOT** one of the responsibilities of an independent contractor?
    a. paying his or her own fees
    b. controlling his or her own hours
    c. paying his or her own taxes
    d. paying franchise fees for the salon _____

22. What is the term for a scheduled meeting with the sole purpose of gathering knowledge about a salon?
    a. information interview
    c. job interview
    b. salon visit
    d. manager consultation
    _____

23. What is a job description?
    a. list of services to be provided in a particular appointment
    b. text in an advertisement describing a job opening
    c. list of an esthetician's specific duties and responsibilities
    d. service description given by the esthetician to a client
    _____

24. What is the umbrella term for methods of increasing contacts and building relationships to further one's career?
    a. incentivizing
    c. contracting
    b. franchising
    d. networking
    _____

25. What are quotas?
    a. percentage of retail sales returned to you as commission
    b. lists of duties and responsibilities related to your job
    c. minimum number of questions you must get right on tests
    d. amounts of goods and services to be sold in a given period of time
    _____

26. What is a written summary of education and work experience that highlights relevant accomplishments and achievements?
    a. quota
    c. commission
    b. job description
    d. resume
    _____

27. What is true of role models?
    a. their behavior and success are worthy of emulation
    b. they represent the opposite of what you want to achieve
    c. they are women hired to showcase clothing, hairstyles, and makeup
    d. every supervisor in every salon is an excellent role model
    _____

28. What is **NOT** among the services commonly offered at resort spas?
    a. skin care
    c. hair and nail services
    b. massage
    d. surgical procedures
    _____

29. What is one tool for writing an effective resume?
    a. avoiding cliched phrases
    b. highlighting personal goals
    c. using vague language
    d. avoiding action or power words
    _____

30. When should you consider writing separate resumes?
    a. when you are trying to hide the fact that you got fired from your last job
    b. when you want to apply for a job without your current employer knowing
    c. when you are applying for different positions with distinct requirements
    d. when you are applying for similar positions at various employers ____

31. What is one technique for considering your audience while writing a resume?
    a. using words to which the reader can relate
    b. using "fancy" language that shows off your intelligence
    c. providing vague information that will force an interviewer to ask questions
    d. leaving out dates so people cannot guess your approximate age ____

32. What is meant by "highlighting your accomplishments" in a resume?
    a. mentioning achievements
    b. identifying how frequently you stay after work to help clean the salon
    c. exaggerating your past salaries
    d. identifying how frequently you were singled out for praise by teachers ____

33. Where in your resume should you mention hobbies that are unrelated to business?
    a. "personal interests" section
    b. employment history
    c. education section
    d. you should not mention these ____

34. What should you **EXCLUDE** from your resume?
    a. employment history
    b. notable accomplishments
    c. description of transferable skills
    d. salary requirements ____

35. What is true about the anxiety you feel when taking a test?
    a. if you feel anxious, you are very likely to fail the test
    b. a certain amount of anxiety may actually help you do better
    c. it is very unusual to experience anxiety when taking a test
    d. if you feel anxious, you should excuse yourself and take the test at a later date ____

36. What is characteristic of a positive attitude toward test-taking?
    a. remembering not to take the test seriously because it's just a test
    b. keeping in mind that individual tests rarely have much impact on final grades
    c. cramming for 24 hours straight immediately before a test
    d. viewing the test as a useful step toward achieving your goals _____

37. What should you do when you encounter options on a test that you know to be incorrect?
    a. eliminate them immediately
    b. assume they reveal "trick questions" and are therefore correct
    c. consider them for a long time
    d. skip the question and go back to it later _____

38. What is the basic question or problem you are being asked to answer and/or solve on a test?
    a. root   c. branch
    b. limb   d. stem _____

39. What does it typically mean if the last word in a stem is *an*?
    a. answer must begin with a consonant
    b. answer must begin with a vowel
    c. all of the answers are likely to be correct
    d. all of the answers are likely to be incorrect _____

40. When should you read the questions in tests that contain long paragraphs of reading followed by several questions?
    a. after you read the paragraph
    b. before you read the paragraph
    c. after you think of the answer
    d. while you read the paragraph _____

41. What should you do on the day of the test?
    a. skip breakfast
    b. leave your watch at home
    c. listen carefully to the examiner's verbal directions
    d. try to answer questions without reading them thoroughly _____

42. What should you do before answering questions on a test?
    a. enter identifying information
    b. read every word of every question
    c. count the number of questions
    d. watch what other students are doing _____

43. When during a test is it appropriate to ask the examiner questions?
    a. when you need help with an answer
    b. when you want to distract the examiner so a friend can cheat
    c. when something is not clear
    d. when you think you can trick the examiner into answering a question ____

44. What should you do if you skip a question?
    a. forget about it and focus solely on the easiest questions
    b. go back later and simply guess at the answer
    c. mark it so you can quickly find it later
    d. cross it out and hand the test in without answering it ____

45. What is the **LEAST** important concern when performing your own trials for the practice exam?
    a. timing
    b. infection control
    c. safety procedures
    d. model's satisfaction with your work ____

CHAPTER 22—THE SKIN CARE BUSINESS

1. When should you confirm that you are in compliance with all local, state, and federal regulations, in order to avoid the risk of violations?
   a. before opening your salon
   b. during your first week of business
   c. during your first month of business
   d. during your first year of business _____

2. Why should you contact local authorities after confirming your ability to own and operate a salon?
   a. to request favorable write-ups in local tourism guides
   b. to investigate necessary business licenses and regulations
   c. to request public financial support
   d. to win favor by offering free services to local authorities _____

3. Whose assistance should you seek out if you do not understand your obligations as a business owner?
   a. marketing specialist and architect
   b. architect and accountant
   c. attorney and accountant
   d. marketing specialist and attorney _____

4. What does OSHA oversee?
   a. efficacy of skin care products   c. product advertising
   b. compliance with tax regulations   d. workplace safety _____

5. What is the purpose of a noncompete clause within an agreement to buy an established salon?
   a. to ensure the seller does not go on to offer similar services to the same market
   b. to ensure the salon has no existing competitors
   c. to void the deal if anyone opens a competing salon within a year
   d. to ensure the buyer will not terminate any current employees _____

6. What procedures should be spelled out in a security checklist?
   a. opening and closing procedures
   b. client-consultation procedures
   c. facial and waxing procedures
   d. greeting and welcoming procedures _____

7. What is a good approach for a business owner to have regarding lapses in insurance coverage?
   a. coverage should never lapse
   b. occasional lapses are not a big deal
   c. coverage is typically unnecessary
   d. insurance should only be purchased when there is a problem _____

8. What key information is supplied by accurate daily reports?
   a. future marketing opportunities
   b. client satisfaction rates
   c. product efficacy fluctuations
   d. gross income and cost of operations _____

9. When answering the phone, how can you let clients know you are eager to serve them?
   a. by rushing them off the phone as fast as possible, because time is money
   b. by telling them questions can only be answered via in-person service
   c. by offering to send an esthetician to their home for the first service
   d. by answering in a sincere, welcoming tone of voice _____

10. What should you **REFRAIN** from doing when using the phone?
    a. being fully attentive to the caller
    b. chewing gum
    c. actively listening to the caller
    d. projecting a positive attitude _____

11. What is the correct term for the money needed to invest in a business?
    a. collateral   c. down payment
    b. lucre   d. capital _____

12. What are consumption supplies?
    a. supplies used in the lunchroom
    b. supplies used to conduct daily business operations
    c. items available for sale to clients
    d. supplies used to build the physical plant of a salon, like lumber _____

13. What are retail supplies?
    a. supplies used in the reception area
    b. supplies used to conduct daily business operations
    c. items available for sale to clients
    d. record-keeping tools like blank sales slips and rolls of receipt paper _____

14. What is **NOT** a characteristic of a corporation?
    a. shared ownership
    b. involvement of stockholders
    c. status as an independent legal entity
    d. ownership limited to one individual _____

15. What is the term for the particular identifying characteristics of an area or population, such as the specific size, age, sex, or ethnicity of its residents?
    a. demographics
    b. quotas
    c. marketing strategies
    d. criteria _____

16. What is an employee manual?
    a. handbook or guide containing data about salon operations
    b. brochure listing businesses with which the salon has professional relationships
    c. list of paid holidays and days the salon will close early
    d. handout with names and contact information of all employees _____

17. What is an example of a fixed cost?
    a. advertising budget
    b. plumbing repair cost
    c. air-conditioning repair cost
    d. rent _____

18. What **BEST** describes a partnership?
    a. multiple stockholders sharing ownership of a business
    b. one person owning a business and another person serving as manger
    c. one person starting a business and then selling it to another person
    d. multiple people sharing ownership of a business _____

19. What term refers to the employees that work for you?
    a. vendors
    b. clients
    c. personnel
    d. constituents _____

20. What is the **PRIMARY** purpose of creating a procedural guide?
    a. standardizing operations
    b. establishing disciplinary policies
    c. weeding out bad employees
    d. relieving managers of responsibility _____

21. What is profit?
    a. total amount of expenses plus revenues
    b. money left after expenses are subtracted from revenues
    c. all salon income prior to expenses
    d. salaries minus tips   ____

22. What is the **MAIN** goal of public relations?
    a. gaining more personal friends
    b. achieving a certain desired behavior
    c. attracting potential new employees
    d. distracting the public from crimes   ____

23. What is revenue?
    a. income generated from selling products and services
    b. amount spent on purchasing products that will be sold to
       clients
    c. total amount of all expenses for which the salon is liable
    d. portion of income set aside for taxes   ____

24. Who generally pays for the utilities an esthetician uses in a
    booth-rental arrangement?
    a. esthetician   c. stockholders
    b. financing company   d. clients   ____

25. What is a business plan?
    a. document outlining a company's beliefs and goals
    b. strategy for understanding key elements in developing
       business
    c. handout given to employees explaining company policies
    d. checklist explaining how procedures are followed   ____

26. What should you do 24 to 48 hours before an appointment with a
    client?
    a. confirm the appointment with the client by phone
    b. prepare your workstation by laying out needed products and
       supplies
    c. turn on the towel warmer and insert fresh linens
    d. wash your hands to ensure cleanliness during the treatment   ____

27. What should you do when leaving phone messages?
    a. remind the client to bring enough money to pay for services
    b. address the client by name
    c. leave a thorough description of all services you expect to
       perform
    d. pretend to be the salon manager   ____

28. What is true of the front desk in a salon or spa?
    a. few customers will have direct interaction with the front desk
    b. only the manager needs to know how the front desk operates
    c. it is the center of business operations in the salon
    d. every esthetician takes a turn working at the front desk   ____

29. What do you gain through education?
    a. compassion for dealing with employees' problems
    b. patience for waiting out slow periods in business
    c. inspiration you need for inventing a successful product
    d. knowledge you need to operate a profitable business   ____

30. When should you become familiar with the basic business principle of accounting?
    a. before you open your business
    b. during your first week in business
    c. during your first month in business
    d. during your first year in business   ____

31. What business type requires the proprietor to bear losses alone?
    a. limited liability corporation   c. partnership
    b. sole proprietorship   d. corporation   ____

32. What sort of person might thrive by operating a sole proprietorship?
    a. collaborative person who enjoys bouncing ideas off others
    b. independent, self-motivated individual who likes to be in charge
    c. risk-averse person who does not mind sharing profits
    d. quiet person who feels uncomfortable giving orders   ____

33. What is a characteristic of someone who might thrive in a partnership?
    a. prefers to do everything instead of delegating tasks
    b. wants to keep all profits instead of sharing them
    c. worries about the risks associated with assuming liability
    d. enjoys the security of working with others   ____

34. When should you learn as much as possible about a prospective partner's ethics and philosophies?
    a. before entering into any binding agreement
    b. before discussing the possibility of going into business together
    c. during the first year of business, so you can see how the person works
    d. after spending your capital on equipment and other necessities   ____

35. What is one of the effects of incorporating?
    a. eliminates the need to pay any type of taxes
    b. requires all investors to be actively involved in managing the company
    c. eliminates the need to obtain government recognition of the business
    d. helps to protect personal assets _____

36. What does a corporation accomplish by issuing stock certificates or shares?
    a. adding members to the board of directors
    b. raising capital
    c. eliminating corporate liability
    d. diversifying corporate investments _____

37. What is a sole proprietorship?
    a. business owned by one person
    b. business owned by two or more people
    c. business owned by stockholders
    d. local business that is part of a larger national chain _____

38. What is the term for business expenses that fluctuate?
    a. fixed costs   c. utility costs
    b. marketing costs   d. variable costs _____

39. What is the right approach for conflicts involving employees?
    a. letting employees work out their own problems
    b. responding quickly and diplomatically
    c. immediately firing any employee involved in a conflict
    d. immediately sending the employee home to "cool off" _____

40. Who do employees typically regard as the leader of the team in the salon?
    a. client
    b. receptionist
    c. manager
    d. most experienced esthetician _____

41. What aspect of employee relations includes active listening?
    a. negative surveillance   c. negative communication
    b. positive surveillance   d. positive communication _____

42. What is an employer's **TOP** financial priority?
    a. payroll   c. rent or mortgage
    b. utilities   d. product vendors _____

43. What costs should you cover for employees to the best of your financial ability?
    a. transportation
    b. meals
    c. benefits
    d. leisure activities
    ____

44. What happens when stockholders buy additional shares of stock?
    a. they diminish the overall value of the corporation
    b. they increase their salaries
    c. their voting power remains unchanged
    d. they increase their ownership interest in the corporation
    ____

45. What type of business is managed by a board of directors?
    a. sole proprietorship
    b. corporation
    c. partnership
    d. booth rental
    ____

46. Why should you require the services of a competent lawyer and tax accountant if you want to form a corporation?
    a. to ensure compliance with complex state rules and regulations
    b. in order to establish tax shelters in which you can hide income
    c. to protect yourself since most companies get sued often
    d. because every business needs a full-time lawyer and tax accountant
    ____

47. What is a benefit of renting a booth or space within an established salon?
    a. booth rental exposes you to every possible business situation
    b. you gain experience by running a business on a small scale
    c. if you succeed in booth rental, you will succeed in anything you try
    d. booth renters usually end up buying the salon after a short period
    ____

48. What are two of the **MOST** important factors when choosing the location of your salon?
    a. product pricing and quality of service
    b. visibility and accessibility
    c. distance from the bank and age of the building
    d. size of the building and quality of its fixtures
    ____

49. What is the term for locating a business close to other businesses that offer different products and/or services?
    a. one-stop shopping
    b. cluster retailing
    c. group marketing
    d. demographic geography
    ____

50. Why is parking a critical element in attracting business?
    a. because employee convenience is always your first priority
    b. safety and convenience are important marketing features
    c. you won't enjoy work if you have to park a long distance away
    d. only people who drive are likely to seek out salon services ____

51. What is a function of the federal agency called the Small Business Administration (SBA)?
    a. ensuring workplace safety
    b. ensuring compliance with employment laws
    c. performing workplace inspections
    d. helping small businesses succeed ____

52. What is true of financial management?
    a. it is your accountant's responsibility, not yours
    b. it is the cornerstone of a successful business plan
    c. no one expects every business owner to know how to manage money
    d. it is the cornerstone of a successful employee handbook ____

53. What helps you learn how to forecast (make predictions) about your business?
    a. achieving five or more years of consistent profitability
    b. maintaining a staff of five or more for at least one year
    c. becoming familiar with the financial affairs of your competitors
    d. becoming familiar with specific costs related to running the business ____

54. What should your dispensary feature in addition to ease of mobility?
    a. soothing paint colors on the wall   c. adequate storage space
    b. high-fashion furniture   d. fluorescent lighting ____

55. What evokes a professional ambience in the salon?
    a. clientele of the salon
    b. style of the salon
    c. neighborhood in which the salon operates
    d. popularity of the salon ____

56. What do you communicate to your employees by setting clear goals and objectives and by acting consistently?
    a. that you are boring and predictable
    b. that you don't want their input
    c. that you are a person of your word
    d. that you will be quick to punish   _____

57. What is the term for items you might offer your employees, such as tickets to educational conferences?
    a. widgets   c. tips
    b. revenues   d. incentives   _____

58. How quickly should you answer the phone in a professional setting?
    a. during the first ring
    b. after about one minute of ringing
    c. you should send all calls to voicemail
    d. within three rings   _____

59. What should you do after asking a caller for permission to put the caller on hold?
    a. immediately put the caller on hold
    b. allow enough time for a response
    c. shout to the person in the salon with whom the caller needs to speak
    d. warn the caller that he or she might be on hold for a long time   _____

60. What is the protocol for missed calls in a professional setting?
    a. every call to a business must be answered immediately
    b. check messages often and respond as quickly as possible
    c. returning these calls is unnecessary because the person will call back
    d. returning calls within a week is sufficiently professional   _____

CHAPTER 23—SELLING PRODUCTS AND SERVICES

1. What is explained in the literature most companies provide for their products?
   a. theory behind their products
   b. details of current litigation
   c. information about which competing products are more effective
   d. information about which competing products are less expensive _____

2. What is the **MAIN** purpose of sales quotas?
   a. to reward the most popular estheticians in the salon
   b. to stimulate growth
   c. to reduce excess stock of retail products
   d. to encourage clients to rebook _____

3. When is it prudent for you to formulate your own sales objectives?
   a. when you think your salon's sales quota system is too aggressive
   b. when you think your salon's sales quota system is too conservative
   c. when your salon does not have a sales quota system
   d. setting sales objectives is never the responsibility of estheticians _____

4. What should you do sometime between 24 hours and one week after a client's salon visit?
   a. place a follow-up phone call
   b. ask the client for a referral to another potential client
   c. send an e-mail asking why the client has not yet returned to the salon
   d. check with the receptionist to see if the client has re-booked yet _____

5. What are benefits of receiving referrals from clients, coworkers, and other people?
   a. enhancing existing clientele and increasing business
   b. being able to increase prices for each new client
   c. being able to completely stop all other promotional activities
   d. decreasing existing clientele by replacing them with new clients _____

6. What is one of the best methods of advertising for a salon?
   a. wearing T-shirts with the salon logo
   b. referrals from current clients
   c. using a keychain with the salon logo
   d. a flashing sign outside the salon _____

7. What client behavior do you encourage by offering clients incentives such as information about upcoming special offers?
   a. constantly asking for discounts
   b. procrastinating
   c. checking out the competition
   d. rebooking   ____

8. When should you find out what the client already knows about his or her own skin?
   a. before trying to educate the client about products or services
   b. after educating the client about products or services
   c. you should always assume the client knows nothing about skin care
   d. you should always assume the client knows everything about skin care   ____

9. When is it appropriate to reveal to the client that you don't know something?
   a. you should always create the impression you know everything
   b. when the client requests information about an unfamiliar subject
   c. when you sense the client wants to "show off" personal knowledge
   d. when the client asks about a service you don't want to perform   ____

10. What is retailing?
    a. practice of encouraging clients to add services to an in-salon treatment
    b. art of recommending and selling products to clients for at-home use
    c. practice of sharing general information about retail products
    d. physical act of ringing up a client's purchase at the register ____

11. What is upselling?
    a. practice of encouraging clients to add services to an in-salon treatment
    b. art of recommending and selling products to clients for at-home use
    c. practice of sharing general information about retail products
    d. physical act of ringing up a client's purchase at the register ____

12. What are consultation skills crucial for accomplishing?
    a. recommending products and services
    b. analyzing product efficacy
    c. complying with safety regulations
    d. adhering to legal requirements   ____

13. What effect do repeat customers have on a business?
    a. deter potential clients from coming into the salon
    b. keep the business flowing
    c. eliminate the need for marketing
    d. eliminate the need for advertising _____

14. Why are estheticians expected to bring clients' attention to sales promotions?
    a. that is the esthetician's role in supporting advertising strategies
    b. supporting advertising strategies is the esthetician's main function
    c. clients want to buy products, not just the treatments they requested
    d. using this technique means the salon doesn't have to pay for advertising _____

15. Whose needs does a successful sales and marketing program meet?
    a. client
    b. esthetician
    c. both client and esthetician
    d. neither client nor esthetician _____

16. What can the esthetician accomplish by learning to recognize the value in selling?
    a. learning how to properly apply recommended products
    b. learning to look at the client as a source of money, not a person
    c. learning to look at products as income rather than as useful tools
    d. moving beyond the negative connotations of selling _____

17. What is one of the esthetician's professional responsibilities?
    a. making the client spend as much money as possible
    b. recommending and providing quality skin care products for clients
    c. getting the client used to buying as many products as possible
    d. selecting retail products based on price, not function _____

18. What do you become once you are educated on the benefits of products and services?
    a. committed to their value
    b. capable of convincing people to make unnecessary purchases
    c. capable of convincing people to spend money irresponsibly
    d. eager to provide them for free _____

19. What are advertisements?
    a. cost-free promotional efforts intended to increase business
    b. artistic treatments of the salon's name used on signs and uniforms
    c. catchy slogans used in newspapers, radio, and television
    d. paid promotional efforts intended to increase business ____

20. What is a benefit of keeping good client records?
    a. serving client needs better
    b. remembering how much to increase prices each visit
    c. identifying the least profitable clients so you can refuse to serve them
    d. creating the illusion of personal service ____

21. What is one possible element of the closing consultation?
    a. analyzing skin type   c. relaxing massage
    b. preparing a home-care program d. hot-towel application ____

22. What is consultative selling?
    a. persuading a client to buy more products or services than planned
    b. telling the client to come back during a future sales promotion
    c. advising clients and recommending the best treatments for them
    d. referring the client to a consultant who can "close" the sale ____

23. What is **NOT** an example of direct marketing?
    a. postcards   c. text messages
    b. coupons   d. upselling ____

24. What term refers to a strategy for how goods and services are bought, sold, and exchanged?
    a. retailing   c. upselling
    b. marketing   d. merchandising ____

25. What term refers to how retail products are displayed in the salon?
    a. upselling   c. merchandising
    b. marketing   d. retailing ____

26. What is promotion?
    a. process of getting the consumer's attention
    b. persuading clients to spend more during a visit than expected
    c. advising clients about the best products for their skin
    d. positioning products in the store so clients see them before leaving ____

27. What is the correct term for free media attention?
    a. advertising
    c. marketing
    b. promotion
    d. publicity   _____

28. What is **NOT** an element of an intake form?
    a. complete client profile
    b. information about client health
    c. data about client skin care habits
    d. credit-card spending limits   _____

29. What is an example of hard selling?
    a. suggesting that a client can come back for a purchase another day
    b. assuring the client that buying a product is not necessary
    c. selling a "hard good" like a product instead of a "soft" one like a service
    d. repeating emphatically why a client should buy a product   _____

30. What can interfere with the relaxation benefit of a treatment?
    a. improperly utilized sales techniques
    b. use of any type of sales technique
    c. the esthetician's touch on the client's skin
    d. soft music playing in the background   _____

31. What is the main criteria for selecting the products and services you recommend to a particular client?
    a. how much that client can spend
    b. benefits for that specific client
    c. whether you think the client will return
    d. whether you think the client will provide referrals   _____

32. When is it recommended that you demonstrate the use of products and treatments?
    a. when you think the client needs an extra push to make a purchase
    b. whenever possible
    c. never
    d. when you think the client can't understand things without help   _____

33. What is **MOST** important for you to know about your products and services?
    a. environmental sustainability
    c. corporate ownership
    b. benefits and features
    d. Consumer Reports rating   _____

34. What can you increase once you gain a comprehensive knowledge of products and services?
    a. retail sales
    b. retail pricing
    c. product efficacy
    d. product popularity

    _____

35. What should you do when faced with an overwhelming amount of information about retail products?
    a. break down product knowledge into manageable categories
    b. select one single product and learn everything there is to know about it
    c. ignore all outside information and rely solely on marketing materials
    d. encourage clients to look into products themselves to determine what they like

    _____

Part 1: Orientation

CHAPTER 1: HISTORY AND CAREER OPPORTUNITIES IN ESTHETICS

1. b	9. a	17. c	25. d	33. b
2. a	10. b	18. d	26. a	34. a
3. c	11. a	19. c	27. a	35. d
4. b	12. c	20. b	28. a	
5. b	13. b	21. a	29. a	
6. b	14. b	22. c	30. b	
7. a	15. c	23. a	31. d	
8. d	16. c	24. d	32. d	

CHAPTER 2: LIFE SKILLS

1. a	9. a	17. c	25. a	33. b
2. b	10. d	18. a	26. b	34. a
3. a	11. a	19. c	27. a	
4. b	12. d	20. a	28. b	
5. c	13. b	21. b	29. c	
6. b	14. b	22. a	30. b	
7. a	15. a	23. c	31. b	
8. a	16. a	24. c	32. a	

CHAPTER 3: YOUR PROFESSIONAL IMAGE

1. b	8. c	15. b	22. b	29. d
2. c	9. d	16. a	23. c	30. d
3. b	10. d	17. a	24. a	31. d
4. d	11. a	18. c	25. b	32. a
5. d	12. b	19. b	26. a	33. b
6. a	13. c	20. a	27. d	34. a
7. b	14. a	21. b	28. b	

CHAPTER 4: COMMUNICATING FOR SUCCESS

1. b	10. b	19. a	28. a	37. d
2. b	11. b	20. b	29. d	38. c
3. c	12. a	21. d	30. c	39. b
4. d	13. a	22. a	31. a	40. a
5. a	14. d	23. d	32. b	41. a
6. b	15. a	24. a	33. d	42. d
7. c	16. d	25. d	34. d	43. b
8. b	17. b	26. b	35. b	44. d
9. d	18. d	27. c	36. b	45. b

Part 2: General Sciences

CHAPTER 5: INFECTION CONTROL: PRINCIPLES AND PRACTICES

1. a	11. d	21. d	31. d	41. c
2. d	12. b	22. a	32. d	42. d
3. a	13. d	23. c	33. b	43. a
4. d	14. a	24. d	34. a	44. b
5. b	15. b	25. b	35. d	45. b
6. d	16. b	26. d	36. c	46. c
7. a	17. b	27. c	37. a	47. d
8. c	18. b	28. d	38. c	48. b
9. b	19. d	29. b	39. b	49. b
10. d	20. d	30. d	40. d	50. b

CHAPTER 6: GENERAL ANATOMY AND PHYSIOLOGY

1. b	13. b	25. d	37. a	49. c
2. b	14. b	26. a	38. d	50. b
3. a	15. a	27. b	39. c	51. a
4. b	16. a	28. d	40. b	52. d
5. c	17. d	29. a	41. a	53. b
6. d	18. d	30. d	42. d	54. d
7. b	19. a	31. d	43. d	55. b
8. c	20. d	32. a	44. b	56. c
9. a	21. b	33. b	45. c	57. a
10. b	22. a	34. a	46. b	58. c
11. c	23. d	35. a	47. d	59. d
12. d	24. b	36. c	48. c	60. a

CHAPTER 7: BASICS OF CHEMISTRY

1. b	9. b	17. d	25. d	33. b
2. a	10. c	18. c	26. b	34. a
3. a	11. c	19. a	27. c	35. b
4. c	12. a	20. b	28. c	36. c
5. a	13. a	21. b	29. d	37. c
6. b	14. d	22. d	30. c	38. c
7. b	15. a	23. a	31. b	39. a
8. d	16. d	24. d	32. c	40. c

CHAPTER 8: BASICS OF ELECTRICITY

1. a	5. b	9. d	13. b	17. b
2. b	6. b	10. a	14. b	18. a
3. c	7. c	11. b	15. b	19. a
4. d	8. a	12. d	16. c	20. c

21. b	25. c	29. d	33. b	37. b
22. b	26. c	30. a	34. d	38. b
23. d	27. a	31. c	35. c	39. c
24. a	28. b	32. c	36. d	40. a

CHAPTER 9: BASICS OF NUTRITION

1. a	10. a	19. b	28. c	37. a
2. b	11. c	20. a	29. a	38. b
3. c	12. b	21. d	30. d	39. d
4. a	13. b	22. c	31. b	40. c
5. b	14. b	23. b	32. b	41. a
6. c	15. b	24. c	33. c	42. b
7. b	16. c	25. c	34. d	43. a
8. a	17. d	26. c	35. d	44. b
9. b	18. c	27. b	36. a	

Part 3: Skin Sciences

CHAPTER 10: PHYSIOLOGY AND HISTOLOGY OF THE SKIN

1. a	14. a	27. a	40. b	53. b
2. a	15. b	28. b	41. a	54. a
3. a	16. b	29. b	42. d	55. a
4. b	17. d	30. d	43. b	56. b
5. d	18. d	31. b	44. d	57. a
6. c	19. a	32. b	45. d	58. c
7. a	20. b	33. a	46. b	59. b
8. b	21. b	34. c	47. a	60. a
9. a	22. b	35. b	48. d	61. c
10. c	23. d	36. c	49. b	62. b
11. b	24. b	37. a	50. b	63. d
12. b	25. d	38. c	51. b	64. a
13. d	26. d	39. a	52. d	65. b

CHAPTER 11: DISORDERS AND DISEASES OF THE SKIN

1. a	10. c	19. b	28. c	37. d
2. b	11. b	20. a	29. d	38. a
3. c	12. b	21. b	30. a	39. d
4. d	13. a	22. b	31. b	40. c
5. a	14. b	23. b	32. c	41. b
6. b	15. c	24. a	33. b	42. d
7. a	16. a	25. a	34. b	43. a
8. d	17. b	26. b	35. d	44. b
9. b	18. d	27. d	36. c	45. d

46. b	54. d	62. d	70. b	78. b
47. d	55. b	63. b	71. b	79. b
48. b	56. d	64. d	72. d	80. a
49. d	57. c	65. a	73. d	81. c
50. d	58. b	66. c	74. a	82. a
51. b	59. c	67. d	75. a	83. b
52. b	60. b	68. d	76. b	84. b
53. a	61. c	69. a	77. b	85. d

CHAPTER 12: SKIN ANALYSIS

1. a	11. c	21. a	31. c	41. d
2. b	12. d	22. d	32. c	42. b
3. b	13. b	23. c	33. c	43. c
4. d	14. a	24. d	34. a	44. b
5. b	15. b	25. a	35. a	45. b
6. d	16. c	26. d	36. c	46. c
7. a	17. d	27. c	37. d	47. d
8. c	18. a	28. a	38. a	48. a
9. c	19. a	29. d	39. a	49. c
10. b	20. a	30. b	40. a	50. b

CHAPTER 13: SKIN CARE PRODUCTS: CHEMISTRY, INGREDIENTS, AND SELECTION

1. a	13. a	25. b	37. c	49. d
2. c	14. c	26. b	38. b	50. d
3. a	15. a	27. b	39. b	51. b
4. a	16. d	28. a	40. c	52. d
5. c	17. b	29. a	41. a	53. a
6. b	18. a	30. d	42. a	54. c
7. c	19. a	31. a	43. c	55. b
8. a	20. b	32. b	44. c	56. a
9. c	21. d	33. a	45. a	57. b
10. c	22. d	34. d	46. d	58. c
11. b	23. b	35. a	47. d	59. d
12. c	24. d	36. a	48. c	60. b

Part 4: Esthetics

CHAPTER 14: THE TREATMENT ROOM

1. a	5. c	9. c	13. b	17. c
2. b	6. b	10. d	14. b	18. a
3. a	7. b	11. a	15. b	19. c
4. d	8. a	12. c	16. c	20. b

21. d	24. a	27. c	30. b	33. a
22. c	25. a	28. c	31. c	34. b
23. c	26. b	29. d	32. b	35. b

CHAPTER 15: FACIAL TREATMENTS

1. a	14. a	27. b	40. b	53. c
2. b	15. d	28. b	41. b	54. d
3. d	16. b	29. c	42. c	55. a
4. d	17. d	30. a	43. b	56. c
5. b	18. b	31. d	44. a	57. b
6. d	19. c	32. c	45. d	58. a
7. b	20. d	33. a	46. b	59. b
8. c	21. b	34. d	47. a	60. d
9. c	22. b	35. b	48. c	61. b
10. a	23. d	36. b	49. a	62. b
11. b	24. c	37. a	50. c	63. c
12. d	25. c	38. a	51. a	64. b
13. c	26. a	39. c	52. b	65. d

CHAPTER 16: FACIAL MASSAGE

1. a	9. c	17. b	25. a	33. c
2. d	10. b	18. a	26. c	34. b
3. c	11. d	19. a	27. d	35. a
4. d	12. a	20. b	28. a	36. a
5. a	13. d	21. c	29. b	37. d
6. b	14. b	22. b	30. a	38. a
7. d	15. a	23. a	31. d	39. c
8. b	16. b	24. d	32. c	40. a

CHAPTER 17: FACIAL MACHINES

1. a	10. c	19. b	28. d	37. d
2. d	11. b	20. b	29. b	38. d
3. b	12. d	21. a	30. b	39. c
4. b	13. a	22. c	31. b	40. a
5. a	14. d	23. d	32. c	41. a
6. a	15. b	24. b	33. c	42. c
7. c	16. d	25. c	34. d	43. d
8. c	17. c	26. b	35. c	44. c
9. a	18. c	27. a	36. d	45. c

CHAPTER 18: HAIR REMOVAL

1. d	4. b	7. d	10. a	13. d
2. c	5. a	8. a	11. b	14. a
3. d	6. c	9. d	12. b	15. c

16. b	23. b	30. a	37. d	44. d
17. a	24. b	31. d	38. d	45. b
18. d	25. d	32. c	39. b	46. d
19. c	26. c	33. d	40. d	47. d
20. b	27. a	34. d	41. d	48. a
21. d	28. d	35. a	42. a	49. d
22. d	29. a	36. c	43. d	

CHAPTER 19: ADVANCED TOPICS AND TREATMENTS

1. a	8. a	15. b	22. b	29. b
2. d	9. d	16. b	23. b	30. b
3. c	10. d	17. c	24. a	31. d
4. d	11. a	18. b	25. d	32. d
5. a	12. c	19. b	26. c	33. a
6. d	13. b	20. a	27. a	34. a
7. d	14. a	21. c	28. d	35. a

CHAPTER 20: THE WORLD OF MAKEUP

1. a	10. c	19. a	28. c	37. a
2. b	11. a	20. c	29. d	38. d
3. a	12. b	21. d	30. d	39. d
4. b	13. d	22. b	31. b	40. d
5. d	14. c	23. d	32. d	41. b
6. d	15. c	24. b	33. a	42. b
7. d	16. d	25. d	34. c	43. d
8. d	17. c	26. d	35. a	44. c
9. a	18. d	27. c	36. a	45. c

Part 5: Business Skills

CHAPTER 21: CAREER PLANNING

1. a	10. c	19. b	28. d	37. a
2. d	11. a	20. c	29. a	38. d
3. d	12. d	21. d	30. c	39. b
4. a	13. d	22. a	31. a	40. b
5. c	14. c	23. c	32. a	41. c
6. c	15. b	24. d	33. d	42. a
7. b	16. b	25. d	34. d	43. c
8. a	17. d	26. d	35. b	44. c
9. b	18. b	27. a	36. d	45. d

CHAPTER 22: THE SKIN CARE BUSINESS

1. a	13. c	25. b	37. a	49. a
2. b	14. d	26. a	38. d	50. b
3. c	15. a	27. b	39. b	51. d
4. d	16. a	28. c	40. c	52. b
5. a	17. d	29. d	41. d	53. d
6. a	18. d	30. a	42. a	54. c
7. a	19. c	31. b	43. c	55. b
8. d	20. a	32. b	44. d	56. c
9. d	21. b	33. d	45. b	57. d
10. b	22. b	34. a	46. a	58. d
11. d	23. a	35. d	47. b	59. b
12. b	24. a	36. b	48. b	60. b

CHAPTER 23: SELLING PRODUCTS AND SERVICES

1. a	8. a	15. c	22. c	29. d
2. b	9. b	16. d	23. d	30. a
3. c	10. b	17. b	24. b	31. b
4. a	11. a	18. a	25. c	32. b
5. a	12. a	19. d	26. a	33. b
6. b	13. b	20. a	27. d	34. a
7. d	14. a	21. b	28. d	35. a

NOTES

NOTES

NOTES

NOTES

NOTES

NOTES

NOTES